Michel Aubin & Philippe Picard

Homoeopathy

A Different Way of Treating
Common Ailments

Translated from the French by
Pat & Robin Campbell

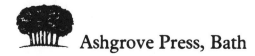

Ashgrove Press, Bath

Published in Great Britain by
ASHGROVE PRESS LIMITED
4 Brassmill Centre, Brassmill Lane
Bath BA1 3JN

and distributed in the USA by
Avery Publishing Group Inc.
350 Thorens Avenue
Garden City Park
New York 11040

Originally published in French

ISBN 1 85398 004 8

This edition first published 1983
Reprinted 1989

Typeset in Plantin by Ann Buchan (Typesetters)
Middlesex
Printed and bound in Great Britain by
Dotesios Printers, Trowbridge, Wiltshire

for Piluche
for Vincent, Laurence and Stéphanie

CONTENTS

PROLOGUE

SCENE 1

'We've brought the child, doctor, because we don't know what to do any more. You looked after our friend's son when he had the same thing and we saw what you did for him—he's so much better now. That's why we've come to you. We've been told homoeopathy is good in some cases and maybe it will work this time. Of course, we don't know. Other people say it's a joke, but we've *seen* it work and we're very upset, so we've come.

'The child is four years old, and for two years now he's suffered continually from colds, tonsilitis and ear infections. He's on antibiotics every fortnight. At first it was only in the winter, now it's all the time—he's all right for a week and then he starts again. He's had his ears syringed several times and he's had his adenoids removed but it hasn't made a scrap of difference. Now our doctor says he's got to have his tonsils out but since his adenoids have already regrown once and the first operation was useless, we don't know what to do.

'When he has a cold there's a whistle in his breathing at night. He coughs a lot and his respiration bothers him. Someone suggested asthmatic bronchitis and we've been advised to take him for a cure.

'On top of that, his appetite is poor. Because he's always ill he can't go to school and the child minder is unwilling to have him any longer, so my wife is going to have to give up work

1

and look after him at home.'

And so on ...

SCENE 2

'Doctor, I've come to see you because I've been told you're good with nerves and I really can't stand the medicines I've being given any longer. I've been told that it's not serious, that there's nothing basically wrong with me and that it's all in the mind—but then I ask myself why for the last five years I've been given tranquillisers, calcium and magnesium, which seem to be the only kind of things that do any good.

'I've already been in hospital for a check-up. There's nothing there, but I suffer just the same. I've been told it will go if I really want to get well, but what I feel is real enough.

'I'm thirty-five. It all began eight years ago after some problems at work. I was given responsibilities which frightened me. I used to get stress symptoms in the mornings before going to the factory. I was given tranquillisers. I felt as if I were better, but I soon found my memory wasn't so good, and then I was tired and I started being impotent. My wife became annoyed—she thought I had a mistress! That unleashed a real crisis, with pains in the stomach and intestines. My X-rays are quite normal, and now, as I say, I've lived for five years on tranquillisers! I can't do without them. I feel I'm living alongside my body. I can't do my work properly any more. I absolutely must find a way out.'

And so on ...

While remaining true to the patients' descriptions, we have deliberately opened this book with two examples which some people might think to be caricatures. Yet, every day, we come across similar situations among our patients. Many readers, whether or not they are doctors, will already have recognised these scenarios. They comprise 80% of current practice.

It seemed important, after having undergone normal hospital training, lived the life of an orthodox doctor and then practised homoeopathy for several years, to bear witness to an undeniable fact: in cases which are incomprehensible to those doctors who are simply technicians in search of observable injury or the physical cause of an illness, and who do not or do not wish to know that there are also imbalances of various regulating mechanisms in a sick person, homoeopathic therapy is especially indicated. The success rate greatly exceeds that occurring through spontaneous remission—which may, incidentally, be observed in all chronic illness and well as in acute illness.

The path we have followed is not unusual: all doctors sensitive to the gap between theory and practice, and who ask themselves some basic medical questions, can do likewise.

One of us was at first a general practitioner in the country, faced every day with real medical emergencies, home-births and minor operations in the surgery, finding a great deal of satisfaction in it all, yet seeing the same patients returning regularly at the same times of the year with the same problems. The other, hospital-trained, practised in general medicine, which put him in touch with various medical bigwigs. He noted with growing astonishment the contrast between their encyclopaedic knowledge and the often disarmingly simple nature of their prescriptions. The higher one rose in the hospital hierarchy, the greater the prevailing scepticism in the efficacy of a wide range of medicines.

Our contact with everyday reality meant that we could not hide behind the white coat, the equipment and the 'hospital image'. We had to find consistent and effective methods of treatment for those cases which we had never come across in hospital but which now accounted for 80% of our patients. How should we confront these illnesses and what weapons should we use?

Chance led us to notice that certain of our patients were cured as a result of homoeopathic treatments prescribed by colleagues. We were continually intrigued by such instances. For us, as for so many, homoeopathy was unknown territory: we had barely heard it mentioned during our student days. At the very most we had a vague recollection of sweeping assertions about this 'quack method' practised by charlatans or fools on credulous patients. Yet these cures were brought about in people whom we knew well and who really had suffered from chronic bronchitis, asthma, eczema and other conditions. We had known them for a long time and, while we had been able to provide relief at times of particular crisis, we had never effected a cure: the crises kept on recurring regularly until finally they exhausted the patient.

We had a private conviction that the solution to these crises lay elsewhere, in this famous area about which people had spoken but which was a mystery to us. Out of intellectual curiosity, and also because we had a taste for therapy, we made enquiries about the colleagues who were using homoeopathic techniques. We were greatly astonished to discover that, far from being chartalans, they were excellent clinicians, observing and studying patients with minute care and then prescribing remedies according to a precise technique which was based on simple, rigorous criteria.

The result of our investigations being initially favourable, we were prompted—in certain individual and carefully defined cases—to try homoeopathic therapy and then afterwards to study the method in a spirit of constructive criticism.

Our first motives for the inquiry were concerned with the advantages the therapy would offer us. Gradually we discovered that this novel approach to the patient allowed us to put his or her specific problems in their general context. In addition, it gave us the possibility of a truly regulatory therapy, whose action was both deep-seated and long-lasting. In this way we were finally able to grasp and properly understand the famous notion of 'constitutional background' which, during our studies, everyone had told us about, but with a dubious smile which left the matter unresolved. What, then, is this 'background' of which everyone talks but for which no one makes any allowance?

We have in us, from birth, in the very structure of our organism, elements which encourage or prohibit the development of this or that illness, for which external events are only a pretext. This holds true even for the development of

4

an infectious disease, which appears at first sight to be a perfect example of an event entirely induced by a chance encounter with that external agent, the microbe. It seems more and more likely that we possess from birth the promise of a line of defence—an 'immunological response', to give it a more technical description—which, for a given pathogen, varies greatly from one person to the next. The rôle of individual heredity in relation to the risk of a given illness becomes ever more glaringly obvious.

It is clear that, after the great era arising from Pasteur's work, during which an 'external' cause was sought for every illness, we are now beginning to appreciate more and more the importance of the individual 'internal' machine, which is innate and which conditions most illnesses. (Jean Hamburger, in *Le mal du siècle* by P. Desgraupes, p. 216.)

Our genetic inheritance determines, without any doubt, the lines of force of our personality. Of course, we no longer believe that the quality of jealousy can be transmitted by heredity, any more than can meticulousness or timidity. But it is likely that two people placed in a given environment, each with their different inheritance, would react differently. (François Lhermitte, *ibidem, idem*, p. 208.)

After our encounter with homoeopathy, our theoretical grasp of the notion of constitutional background remained almost as vague as before, but in practical terms we were finally able to study the mode of reaction of each of our patients; once we had recognised this individuality, we could react effectively by modifying our prescription accordingly.

Everyone knows that, in current practice, interpreting improvement is a relative matter, and everyone knows about the success of 'healers' and charlatans of all shades. We tried to be rational, to observe, to compare and to be objectively critical. Some of the cures we obtained were quasi-miraculous, quite inexplicable: we could not reproduce them and so concluded that we had achieved a simple placebo effect. Others, however, were reproducible, under the same conditions and with all patients in the same way, whatever their age or social background. This fact was enough, by itself, for us to recognise and admit that homoeopathy was a well founded therapy. Only much later, irritated by the objections and systematic refusal of our colleagues to look open-mindedly at our clinical observations, were we led to take note of experimental work done under laboratory conditions, and from there to undertake our own experiments to show the very real pharmacological effects of homoeopathic remedies on animals.

Having practised homoeopathy for a number of years (fifteen in one case, twenty in the other), we became more and more firmly persuaded of the benefit of this therapy, both in current medical practice and in fundamental research. Additionally, and not least amongst its advantages, we have become convinced that it can play a leading rôle socially and economically in changing the world's conception of what constitutes a health problem.

Now that we have established what we were sure of, and then having submitted it to lengthy and fundamental criticism, we feel bound to offer our testimony in favour of homoeopathy. We feel that doctors, students, pharmacists and patients should be told without delay of the scope of this method, and given details of its limitations and conundrums as well as its great potential. Such is the aim of this book which, as well as being a testament, is meant to open up discussion.

We are sufficiently realistic, however, not to take it for granted that homoeopathy may one day be in the forefront of medical teaching. There are too many obstacles to prevent this, arising both from the 'fringe' homoeopaths who still exist and from certain branches of officialdom: these amateurs, on the one hand, and defenders of hallowed ground on the other, seem to be becoming more and more numerous. However, we are convinced that all doctors should be aware of the usefulness and reality of homoeopathic practice so that they may, in full knowledge of the facts, make a therapeutic choice to the benefit of their patients.

We are defending a method which is simple in both theory and practice. The strict use of the technique is not, we know, currently practised by the majority of doctors who call themselves homoeopaths, but its simplicity should compel recognition in spite of the hostile attitude which is sometimes found even in homoeopathic circles.

We want this testimony to be quite free of polemic- —polemic would be only too easy, given the often contradictory schools of thought which are to be found in the medical profession. Moreover, we have tried to be careful not to be guilty of that eccentricity which has always irritated us in books devoted to so-called 'natural' medicine, into smugness and an absence of the constructive critical faculty, wrong interpretation due to lack of knowledge of the scientific reality, risky extrapolation, hazily speculative theorising and, lastly, stultifying compartmentalisation.

We hope that our readers will be aware of the constant concern which motivates us: the search for a balance between the known and the unknown.

CHAPTER I

Doctor, Patient and Medicine

Medicine is today in a state of flux—an obvious enough statement to make. To be aware of it one has only to open a newspaper, turn on the television or run one's eye along the library shelves: one is constantly confronted by one or other of the critical questions being asked by medical practitioners, users of the health service, sociologists, politicians and those authorities whose job it is to instil order in a very complicated subject.

A diminishing band of people think that everything is going well and that it is senseless to raise such issues. However, another group considers that everything is going wrong, and that only a radical change can bring about the introduction of a coherent health policy—but they can't agree on what sort of change should be introduced.

What has happened to bring us to this point? The answer is simple. The power of medicine, its hold on our everyday life and the constant glorification of its results have been magnified out of all proportion, so that, after a period of self-satisfied admiration and acceptance, they have been rejected in a way that could easily have been foreseen. Delusion has followed euphoria. Perhaps this swing will eventually settle down, leaving us at a sensible balance-point between these two opposite and apparently mutually incompatible extremes.

The problem is further confounded by the fact that no two people define simple words like 'medicine', 'doctor', 'illness'

8

and 'patient' in the same way. Everyone extends or limits the meaning of the terms to their own advantage.

What is an illness?

An illness is well defined, always similar and attached to a specific cause, say some. A reactive mode causing the interaction of multiple agents against a more or less favourable constitutional background, say others. It is an entity, but there are nuances, as Funck-Brentano said: there are 'illnesses in uniform and illnesses in hooded cloaks'. The illness should be seen as an entity which is external to the patient and can be known only through its objectively measured symptoms. Illness is a modification of the normal behaviour of a subject who has become ill and who lives through the illness in his or her own way—in this case it can be appreciated only by paying close attention to the subjective symptoms which give it its own 'fingerprint'. Illness can and must be isolated and studied *per se*. Illness has no existence of its own: there are only ill people.

On the one hand, then, in this jumble of ideas we see constant reductionism, striving to be analytic and scientific, and desperately determined to stay in the realm of the measurable and reproducible. On the other, there is unlimited extension, often degenerating into totally loose thinking and guesswork. On both sides, every school of thought is divided into many sub-schools, each of which thinks that it alone holds the key to the truth.

What is a patient?

Someone who has a clearly defined illness? Someone who feels ill? A number in a bed? A 'gall bladder' or a 'stomach', as one sometimes hears patients described in hospitals? A unique person, unlike any other? A person who must without protest hear his medical sentence passed? Someone who has a right to health? The one who has to submit or the one who, in the last resort, is sole arbiter of the decision to be taken?

What is medicine? In which areas does it apply?

The search for organic disorder, or even functional disease, so long as it is measurable, objectified and clearly labelled? An ideology, a concept of life, of health, of illness determined by a collection of doctors who decide that 'that and that alone' is medicine? A power, the notorious 'medical power' which is currently contested? An instrument of power, as certain politicians seem to think and to which others, not yet in power, themselves object? A basic science following exact rules from which it may not with impunity depart? An art, allowing doctors to fend for themselves when faced with their patients, inventing treatments afresh each time, according to the inspiration of the moment?

What is a doctor?
A technician, a dispenser of care? Someone who knows everything about everything, or who knows nothing but dabbles in everything? Someone who 'punishes' by forcibly inflicting diets, dangerous drugs, radiotherapy or surgical mutilation? Someone who helps and loves, and who alleviates suffering? Someone who wishes to dominate patients? Someone who wants to keep them in a state of dependence? Someone who wants to help them become responsible for their own health? Someone who makes money out of them and exploits them, or someone who is devoted to them?

We are faced with an endless variety of images, judgements and assertions, based sometimes on the rational, sometimes on the poorly mastered irrational. There are so many uncertainties. It is a strange game in which every player plays according to their own rules, unaware of or ridiculing other peoples'; it is a rat-race in which anything goes and where the primary aim is 'victory' over the other person. The problem is hopelessly involved, and becomes ever more insoluble.

There is a constant shift of emphasis between the opinions of certain centres of conservative medical opinion, others better integrated into the contemporary realities, and yet others who are more idealistic and geared towards the future, while the distances between the viewpoints of patients are similarly great. Some people are still convinced that conventional medicine is all-powerful, while others vigorously reject it in favour of 'natural' therapies.

These disagreements create an astonishing number of problems which are reflected in everyday medical practice. The patient's appeal and the doctor's response both fall on deaf ears, leading to more or less open rebellion by the patient and more or less cynical rejection by the doctor. The doctor is no longer sure just what to expect from the patient, and doesn't appreciate the real meaning of his or her appeal. Patients are no longer very sure just what a doctor can or ought to do for them. General confusion reigns, and as a result the realm of health care is extended in ways which are both unforeseen and hard to control. By its very scale this problem has become one of the most worrying of our time, particularly in the economic sphere.

MEDICINE ADRIFT

The job of medicine is twofold: to study illnesses and to look after patients. However, by a strange paradox which only confuses the issue, patients need not necessarily be suffering from an illness. Illness has gradually emerged from the realm of superstition and become an object of study to which people have tried to apply the scientific method. There is a very basic question to be answered: is medicine a science? *Can* it be a science?

P. Guicheney has rightly said: 'Medical science *per se* does not exist. It is a composite thing with at least two main constituent groups: basic sciences and clinical sciences.'

Straightaway there arises a major problem, one which will confront us for as long as we refuse to recognise and resolve it. What should be the respective rôles of basic science and clinical science? In practice, this question is posed although not outright in a rather different way: who, the theoretical scientist or the clinical scientist, is going to dominate in the world of medicine, given that both are convinced they are right? The question has been politicised—in the derogatory sense of that

11

term—and the problem has thereby become more insidious.

Clinical medicine, based on the minute observation of symptoms and their logical classification, reached the height of its influence in the nineteenth century, yet even then it never led to effective therapy. Older doctors will undoubtedly recall medical treatises which, with great precision and in minute detail, described for page after page the symptoms and clinical forms of every conceivable illness, only to conclude each chapter with a painfully thin and banal paragraph describing therapy.

Over the last fifty years the successive and related discoveries of numerous drugs and the development of more and more specific techniques, stemming from the continuous progress of the basic sciences, have seemed to make even the most optimistic dreams legitimate. But as J. P. Escande has pointed out, 'People thought that the progress of biology would give birth to a radically new form of medical practice, one imbued with science. It is believed today that those people were mistaken, that they went too far.' However, this doesn't prevent people from according the basic sciences privileged status, from favouring specific research, from developing ever more sophisticated techniques. And meanwhile they continue to ignore or forget the problems which doctors in practice confront every day, and in the face of which they must respond almost entirely by the use of improvisation. For one thing they are faced with illnesses which they never encountered during hospital training, even if only a straightforward case of measles, chickenpox or shingles. For another, doctors see patients who complain of strange problems which for want of training they simply do not understand. These polymorphous disorders bear no relation to the objective, well classified, recognisable illnesses they have studied. Every day patients come to complain of insomnia, tiredness, vertigo, headaches, intestinal problems and many others; and the doctor doesn't know what to do about them.

Yet—alas for their useless knowledge!—most doctors will seldom if ever be called upon to take the decision to operate on a congenital cardiac malformation, with all types of which, down to the rarest, they are familiar, as well as the very latest techniques as applied in such and such ultraspecialised hospital. Doctors also know the precise pharmacological action of the most modern and most powerful drugs, but are hardly ever called upon to prescribe them except for benign conditions—in such cases the drugs are not only manifestly useless but may also have considerable adverse side-effects. Sometimes, without in any way wishing to, doctors themselves contribute to the general lack of health—a situation which is patently absurd!

Countless trivial complaints are treated with powerful antibiotics. People who are suffering from minor neuroses or who are simply unhappy are dosed with tranquillisers or sedatives. All this comes about because excessive credence is given to the methods which medicine has at its disposal, and through ignorance or misunderstanding of the real needs of health. The situation is the logical end-product of a system of medical education which is poorly adapted to real needs and which places excessive weight on the basic sciences, which are indispensable only to professional researchers, while casting scornfully aside the teachings of modern pathology.

The medical profession is so structured that, as is generally agreed, there is a growing disparity between the patients seen by the general practitioner and those encountered in the university and teaching hospitals. As Lagache and Hoerni note in an article in the *Bordeaux Médical*:

> The patients a medical student sees during his time at teaching hospital no longer have very much in common with those he will see as a general practitioner. The development of medicine and the evolution of the hospital structure, particularly that of the teaching hospitals, are responsible for increasing selectivity in the admission of patients to the places where the basic medical training is given. Because the patients are sifted before being admitted, they no longer provide typical examples of pathology. In these hospitals

most of the teachers operate full-time: they have no experience of private practice and are sometimes unaware that the ranges of patients they deal with is only a fraction of the breadth of that seen by a general practitioner.

To back up their claim Lagache and Hoerni cite a number of studies, especially those by John Fry, a general practitioner in the London suburbs, who states from experience: 'Serious, potentially fatal illnesses represent only 5% of the total number of patients seen in twenty years of practice.' Other studies carried out in Norway, the United States and France, confirm this. An investigation carried out by Lagache and Hoerni and their pupils brought the following conclusions in relation to cancer, their specialisation:

Cancer patients represent only 1-2% of all those seen by the general practitioner ... Breast and uterine cancer in women, lung cancer and cancers of the upper respiratory tract in men, and cancer of the oesophagus in both sexes may quite regularly be encountered by the general practitioner, but other forms of cancer really are rare. He is likely to see one or two cases of leukemia in ten years and only a few doctors will see a nephrobalastoma in a child during thirty or forty years' practice.

These general points will be familiar to anyone concerned with health matters and the glaring inadequacy of medicine to cope with the realities of medical practice. Nevertheless, do they constitute sufficient reason to throw everything overboard and adopt, as common currency, the ideas put forward by Ivan Illich in his book, *Medical Nemesis?* These virulent ideas were readily taken up by the popular press and media as a novelty; but they had long been known to doctors familiar with the theses proposed by the zealous partisans of 'parallel medicine' or by the 'anti-doctors'—who were around long before this term was coined. One of us actually heard an 'anti-doctor' say, in all seriousness and strictly in accordance with his own system of logic: 'Homoeopathy will rise only from the corpses of the medical faculties.'

14

Remarks of this sort, especially those from Illich, have always irritated us—indeed, disgusted us—by their illogical excess. They are simply the expression of a deeply, half-baked wish to change one doctrine for another by violent means. Either these people have not studied the problem (which doesn't seem to be Illich's case) or else they are parodying what might happen were they to be taken seriously. However, as Pierre Vianson-Ponté said in the enthralling book which he wrote with Leon Schwarzenberg shortly before his death:

> When Illich maintains that, in our profit-oriented consumer society, medicalisation has reached excessive proportions and hides very real dangers, is he entirely wrong? When he claims that the development of the medical institution, which he sees as anti-life, has a bad influence on health, is he completely mistaken? To say that he goes too far, that he throws the baby out with the bath water in preaching against medical progress—even praising the dark ages and the medicine of the 'noble savage'—is to take the soft option of rebutting everything he says.

In this sort of discussion, often pushed to the extremes, the problem is never stated accurately, always in fallacious terms. Who would dare deny that recent medical research has enabled tubercular meningitis to be cured, that significant progress has been made in the treatment of leukemia, that some cancer patients, thanks to a combination of new techniques, are granted an increasingly long survival time? Is that any reason to draw a veil over everything *else* that is going on in the medical field and to deny other therapies which are gentler and better adapted to sickness in general?

A DOCTOR LOOKS FOR THE RIGHT ROAD

What of the doctor in all this? Faced with a mass of medical technology which he can't use, uniformed in the universities of the kind of patients he is going to encounter in his daily round, he is put in an uncomfortable position. What is his rôle? What

15

has he been trained for? Can he fulfil the demands of the patients in his practice? Will working merely as a technician, applying the rules he has learned—observation, diagnosis and treatment—satisfy him? If so, the number of possible scenarios will be strictly limited.

First Scenario: The doctor sends the patient to a specialist, who makes the diagnosis which he himself cannot for lack of technical equipment.

Second Scenario: The doctor sends the patient to hospital for treatment which, because of the strict 'etiquette' involved, cannot be given at home. F. Caviglioni put it this way in an article in the *Nouvel Observateur* newspaper: 'Nowadays, thanks to the progress which medicine has made, a patient is no longer someone who can look after himself. He has to be taken into reception and then despatched to various locations.' Behind this wry statement lies a sad truth.

Two further scenarios are somewhat less spectacular:

Third Scenario: The doctor is able to diagnose a number of illnesses which he can treat in model fashion according to the rules he learned at medical school: diabetes and angina, for instance. However, these illnesses, which form the basis of the practice, are relatively rare.

Fourth Scenario: The doctor comes across the whole gamut of benign illnesses, his sole knowledge of which is from books, for he has never had the opportunity to observe a real case. However, he remains calm: he knows that, by definition, they will get better of their own accord and that not only is treatment easy but it also has little effect—one can even abjure treatment altogether, he was told when he was a student. However, very soon he discovers that things are not really like that, especially in the matter of diagnosis. The rash on a child's skin bears only a slight resemblance to what he was shown on a slide. Measles? German measles? An allergy? Food poisoning? He is uncertain and embarrassed. A temperature of 40°C (104°F) with no accompanying symptoms could indicate almost anything. One has to wait and watch the patient in order to produce a diagnosis; but the patient's relations and the patient himself are not content just to wait without treatment, any more than they are prepared to allow the illness to run its course. The cure must be quick— preferably instantaneous! The doctor does not have the right to make a mistake, but the patient has the right to as rapid a cure as possible—and so the doctor is forced to act which means prescribing powerful medicines in order to cover himself, through fear of a wrong diagnosis and to please the patient, as well as through failure to recognise that there are other therapies.

That leaves the *Fifth Scenario*, the one which is most often encountered. In addition to those patients who allow the doctor to practise his profession as he has been taught, there are all the others whom he must receive, listen to and treat, those who care nothing for the technicalities of medicine and who, in the absence of a clearcut diagnosis, are content just to be understood and cared for. They form 80% of the total. The doctor's only answer is to treat them as individuals, studying each case as a whole.

'For illnesses which are not clear-cut,' wrote M. Balint, 'for psychosomatic and functional conditions and for organic conditions which have become chronic or terminal, only treatment which is centred on the patient rather than on the illness will prove effective.' As O. Rossowsky said in a supplement of the *Nouvel Observateur* newspaper, devoted to health: 'In promoting only the interests of biological research and acute cases, those who administer the system as it is now constituted end by forgetting one particular element: man.' And, later in the same article: 'Only medicine dealing in a spectacular way with acute cases receives enough backing. The rest of the medical system is so structured that it simply selects and provides the "necessary subjects".' In the same issue Norbert Bensaïd added:

Faced with the grossly technical nature of what is learned at medical school, and with clinical training concerned exclusively with hospital-oriented pathology and differing in every way from daily practice, the student runs the risk, as the young teacher Béatrice Le François has put it, of 'wavering between pseudo-commonsense, which one knows

17

can only be the reflection of personal prejudices he has acquired in good faith, and the temptation of imitating real, proper medicine by prescribing uselessly and ordering senseless investigations. He is given the choice between becoming a technician or believing that without technology he will be like a doctor from a previous age.'

Indeed, this is more or less what happens, but why dictate a single course? Why block off other possibilities? Why continue to operate this absurd blackmail? If a doctor becomes a technician and venerates what, at the time, is held to be sacrosanct, then he is integrated into the medical fraternity and gains credence; but if he wants to act otherwise he downgrades himself and ultimately excludes himself from the fraternity. Why can a doctor not be simultaneously a technician and a so-called old-fashioned doctor, an individual who unites in himself two cultures which have become separate through rejection, on the one hand, and voluntary apathy, on the other? In his excellent book, *What Is a Doctor?* (*Qu est-ce que le médecin?*), P. Guicheney has been able, as the result of an enquiry carried out among both patients and doctors, to establish the various rôles which patients expect their doctor to play, and the type of relationship they hope to have with him. According to Guicheney's conclusions, this relationship should work on three levels: the anatomical, the psychological and the social. 'The doctor must, in future, consider all three aspects of the patient: body, person and holder of social rights.' To do this the doctor has, on the one hand, to put into operation the technique he has learned, and on the other to listen attentively.

In so doing he moves from the realm of science to that of technique or art which, according to *Robert* [*Dictionnaire de la langue française*] is the sum of the means, the set procedures, which lead to an end. Confronted by his patient, the doctor will work out a particular method of prceeding, bearing in mind what he knows of the patient, his previous history and his heredity. He has continually to compromise between the possible, the desirable and the scientifically necessary.

The doctor has to be fully familiar with the technique to which he must resort in any particular case where its strict application is necessary. In an emergency, such as a ruptured ectopic pregnancy or a pulmonary embolism, he carries out certain actions almost automatically, by reflex, forgetting for the moment that he is dealing with a person who is ill, sometimes even deliberately making the situation abstract so as to avoid any emotional factors which might slow down the operation.

On the other hand, faced with a medical decision concerning something like a stone in the bladder or a stomach ulcer, there is no question of considering the sick person in the abstract, nor the manner in which this apparently localised illness has come about, nor yet the relationship between his condition and any psychological or behavioural problems he may have. Nor can the family or social background of the patient be ignored, for medical and surgical decisions must often be taken in line with certain conditions quite external to the patient himself.

Every medical decision has to be tailored to the patient. This perfectly obvious fact is frequently stated indeed, too frequently for it ever to be put into practice. There is another point on which it is right to insist: every such decision depends also on the personality of the doctor who makes it or who helps the patient to make it. However much it expresses the reality of the situation, this attitude is not often referred to by the medical fraternity which, while it wishes to recognise (although it does not always succeed) the individual nature of the patient, is much less prepared to give equal recognition to the individual nature of the doctor. Instead, the establishment tries to turn out doctors who are all the same and readily interchangeable. This is certainly true at the basic level of training: fame, together with uncontested and indeed incontestable authority, is reserved to the few. In seeking to negate the important rôle which the doctor's personality plays in the job of medicine, trying increasingly hard to reduce therapy to a purely technical act, the majority of those in authority in the medical profession are responding more or less consciously to the wishes of the various technocrats in their structural plans for medicine.

Yet, as P. Guicheney points out, a doctor's choice of action is always affected by cultural influences: 'The student, the doctor and the researcher are imbued with a microculture; what is true of general medical thought is true of each doctor in particular ... The numerous options on offer—allopathy in its various manifestations, homoeopathy, acupuncture, naturopathy, psychosomatics, and so forth—have all been elaborated with reference to a particular order.' This microculture may or may not be in accord with the general culture of the time, for one can frequently see, in many different periods and under a variety of circumstances, cultural modifications allowing the acceptance at a particular point in time of microcultures more generally considered to be on the fringe, only for them to be rejected again later.

In daily medical practice, every doctor relies simultaneously on on medical science and on an individual perception of what medicine is. Medical science forms a reassuring and solid system of reference. The concept of the practice of medicine permits a true dialogue with the patient, and this in turn leads to an improvement in the doctor's awareness and understanding of the symptoms and also in the explanation which he gives to the patient. This dialogue relates to a common cultural background, which in reality is far too complex to be reduced to the domination of any ideology imposed from within a system, defining its own laws and arbitrarily choosing its own criteria. The practical model conceived by the doctor is only a particular form which enables him, using a certain view of medicine, to group symptoms according to a particular system of logic and as a result draw conclusions as to a suitable course of action. Alongside the model suggested and approved by the current medical system, there may be other models which work just as well and in some cases considerably better.

THE PATIENT WHO NO LONGER
KNOWS WHICH DOCTOR TO TRUST

What happens to the patient in all this? What are his expectations? What are his demands?

His paramount wish is that he be looked after; that is to say, examined, listened to and understood. He wants to know what he's got and what he can do or what can be done for him. These are apparently simple demands, yet more often than not they are hard to meet.

The relationship between doctor and patient is in practice an ambivalent one, and the links which are established are often not expressed at all clearly or accurately by the two parties. Primarily based on emotion, the relationship can transform very quickly, passing from total confidence to profound distrust or biting criticism. Nor, curiously enough, is there any direct or logical link between the relationship and the success or failure of the therapeutic measures adopted.

We all have patients who thank us or sing our praises when our rôle has been minimal or nonexistent. Others part from us rancorously when we have acted in a perfectly adequate manner to protect the patient from potential dangers of which he was not even aware.

For the patient, medicine is a world apart: he can have only an outsider's view of it. Just as well, say some; more's the pity, say others. He doesn't have any active part to play; and no 'open-door' policy in hospitals is going to alter that situation very much, for too many other factors are involved. He penetrates the medical world only occasionally, because he needs to or because he wants to, and it is rare for him to do so without fear. Medicine arouses fear by its complex equipment, its apparent omnipotence and its carefully conserved air of mystery. It terrifies by its quasi-absolute power over the patient's body and by the verdicts, against which there is apparently no appeal, which from time to time it is led to pronounce. This apprehension, felt and shown to a greater or lesser degree, keeps the patient in a state of dependence, and this can lead to aggressive reactions which he makes no effort to hide, especially when he is not ill.

Medicine is, or wishes to be, completely scientific—we have already noted and expressed our regret about this. Medicine uses complicated pieces of equipment whose results the patient cannot decipher. For his part, the doctor often uses terms which need to be translated into everyday language before the patient can hope to understand them. On top of this, the doctor wants to know things: he *needs* to know things, and so he asks very specific questions; the effect is sometimes rather like an interrogation. The answers have to be phrased clearly and without ambiguity, so that they may be understood, accepted and recorded. It is salutary to observe the embarrassment of certain patients with a restricted vocabulary who are unused to dealing with medical terminology. Quite suddenly they are unable—or do not dare—to recount the manner of their suffering. From the outset of the consultation they seek to dress up their own approximate diagnosis of their illness with a 'learned' name; 'It's my gall bladder' or 'It's my nerves.' Surrendering their own free will in the face of medical techniques and judgements, they respectfully or triumphantly place on the doctor's desk the X-rays or analyses which, they are convinced, will indicate better than any description on their part what is wrong with them. Faced with a doctor who is unaware of the situation or hasn't the time to listen, they dare not open their mouths. Yet in the waiting-room, or at home, or at the shops or the market or the hairdresser's, what a plethora of detailed symptoms they describe!

But this verbal feast dries up at the doctor's door, finding only a very poor expression in a meagre few words borrowed, if at all possible, from the medical canon. Agreement is thus reached on 'a gall bladder' or 'a stomach' or 'too much fat in the blood'. The patient stands there with his prescription and the results of his tests, and keeps saying 'You must look at these', and *fails to describe his symptoms*. Some patients, it is true, are satisfied with this sort of diagnosis. Their illness has been named—it really exists. Now they know what is the matter with them, and they feel reassured. The doctor, too, is satisfied, and so the pair of them are committed, easily and often unconsciously, to a superficial relationship which will last for a long time and cost a lot of taxpayer's money for regular consultations, medicines and routine tests.

Who is responsible for this? The doctor who practises as he has been taught? But he has found an abnormality and corrected it: is that not his function? The patient who wouldn't or couldn't express himself? But his failure to describe how he feels has not been too important, surely, since he was fortunate enough to come across a good doctor who apparently found out right away what was the matter: it could have been much worse.

In fact, neither of them is to blame: it is the perversion of medicine induced by the system that has trapped these two without either being aware of it.

Conversely, some patients feel let down and frustrated: they wanted to talk and be listened to. They maintain that what they had to say has been bypassed, that they have been processed as swiftly as possible, and labelled so that they could be put into some convenient pigeonhole and there abandoned. Some note that, while the doctor may ask questions, he gives scant attention to the replies, and starts the next question before the patient has finished answering the first. They are perfectly aware that the medical dialogue between them takes place only according to certain rules imposed by the doctor, the arbiter of the game, and that no other form of exchange is possible. The doctor, representing 'medicine', is there to diagnose an illness and not to waste his time listening to useless detail. As far as he is concerned, illness can be expressed only in terms of clear, precise, readily recognisable symptoms: the rest is so much verbiage and of no interest. The patient is not really expected to want to talk. Of course, one listens to him a bit, but not for long. If the conversation veers too far from medical logic, if it becomes nonsignificant and uninteresting, then one turns it more into an interrogation by asking 'real' questions—that is, ones designed to extract precise information about the nature of the problem. But, as M. Balint has it, 'when one asks questions one gets answers and nothing more'.

In practice, this method nearly always enables one to find *something*, for there is nearly always an anomaly somewhere. The real difficulty arises if one has to judge the importance or significance of this anomaly, but fortunately this problem doesn't occur most of the time. A diagnosis is made and the interview is closed with the issue of a prescription. The patient feels let down, won't accept it, goes to see another doctor, then another and yet another, until he is truly listened to and properly taken in hand as an individual patient.

For the patient, the doctor is clearly the representative of 'medicine'. He knows the technical rules and can operate them, but he is also the embodiment of quite another form of knowledge, which is much wider-ranging and whose limits are ill defined. The doctor is not only 'the one who is supposed to know' but also the one who is supposed to be able to act.

Except in extremely urgent cases the patient chooses his doctor, and this choice is never a haphazard one; but the patient makes it according to his own personal criteria rather than scientific ones. He finds out, for instance, what sort of practice a doctor has and about his character, his bedside manner and the sort of things he prescribes. Every doctor possesses an 'aura', according to what he is or appears to be, which draws a certain kind of patient. In his book *Changing Death (Changer la mort)*, Léon Schwarzenberg suggests, only half-jokingly, the setting-up of a guide to doctors and hospitals, a sort of medical *Michelin Guide* which would award the doctors stars. This would be easy enough to do if doctors were simply mechanics or technicians. But we know—and so, incidentally, does Schwarzenberg—that although technique is an essential of good medicine it is only one of numerous elements, many subjective, which are involved when we seek to define what makes a good doctor. A good doctor—but for whom and in what context? The human qualities complement the technical ones, but are much harder to pin down.

An individual's knowledge can only be specialist knowledge, in a chosen field, and with inevitable gaps and weaknesses; it is most important for every doctor to be aware of this. We have seen that the doctor-patient relationship fits into a climate of opinion based on a number of set ideas, and this consensus, even if sometimes misleading, allows good relations to be established rapidly. If there is a fair degree of understanding, then the relationship continues; otherwise, sooner or later, it ceases, either because the patient goes to consult another doctor or else because the doctor himself suggests or implies that it would be better if the patient were to seek treatment else-where—or even that he can go hang! This attitude isn't usually so clearly expressed, and may well be hidden behind requests for consultations with various specialists or for biological or X-ray examinations that have no other purpose than to bolster up a failing relationship.

In addition to the technical setting-in-motion of processes designed to substantiate (or otherwise) the presence of an illness, there is always an input based on the state of the relationship and this is composed of imponderables. The purely ideological option of limiting oneself to the almost obsessional search for a discernible malady has brought into being a super technology which calls upon more and more complex machinery and gives rise to 'superspecialists in sub-specialisations', who limit their activity to the study of one tiny portion of the individual.

François Laplantine has noted that 'the modern mentality, in which each sphere of knowledge is treated as unrelated to the others, in medical terms separates the psychic from the organic and then, supposedly in the name of progress, divides the human organism up into a multiplicity of areas', and 'cultural differences, lack of symmetry, the great divide between doctor and patient, are becoming much more marked these days ... The gulf between the symbolic language of the patient, who is by nature not scientific but affective, and the doctor's hieroglyphic response has increased.'

The patient often feels fragmented, dissected. While in particular instances he may accept this, in general he cannot feel happy about it, particularly as this technological abuse, this 'technicalistic perversion of medicine' as J. P. Escande puts it, leads necessarily to demands for further examinations and to the excessive consumption of prescribed medication whose side-effects can prove more and more troublesome.

Weary of being treated as objects, increasingly disgusted by large quantities of drugs (one sees patients who daily swallow eighteen to twenty tablets, pills or capsules with a variety of names for a variety of ailments), patients are turning in ever increasing numbers to simple therapies and to people

25

who are prepared to hear them out and to talk in their own language, so-called 'parallel' or 'unofficial' doctors, psychologists and psychiatrists, and even faith-healers and quacks. They thereby run all the risks inherent in a desire to trust only in Mother Nature.

WHAT IS TO BE DONE?

The inevitable conclusion is that classical, scientific medicine is unable to answer most of the questions asked of it. This does not mean that we should reject or abandon the positive things which it has brought us. But we feel obliged to say that there are other answers, that there are *other methods of treatment* which are, sadly, too little known and used. An artificially high value has been placed on some methods of treatment which alone are considered effective, and this situation cannot be allowed to continue. It is vital that doctors learn of the existence of the alternatives as part either of their theoretical or practical training. Patients, too, should have clear precise knowledge, free from myth, about what is available.

J. P. Escande points up the situation with some verve:

The concept that many of those involved have of medicine is erroneous because it is the product of a tragic error. It was thought that progress in biology would lead to the birth of a new sort of thoroughly scientific medical practice. Today it seems that it was a mistake to go so far. Medical practice today remains pretty much as it was yesterday and the day before, although with the difference that the doctor can think things out more logically in advance and so draw more efficient therapeutic conclusions. But the basic structure of the medical act stays the same. Let me make a comparison. No one questions the advantages of a jet aircraft; yet every day trains and small propeller aircraft render valuable service. Would you travel a hundred miles by jumbo jet? It would be a long and costly way of making the journey. Yet in medicine, increasingly, the impressive tools that are available are used—to ill effect. It is a mistaken trend which consumes fabulous sums of money—which are more and more difficult to raise—without bringing any new benefits to the patient.

There are many ways of approaching an illness, understanding it, and treating it. Why is each not used when it is applicable, for no single one excludes any of the others? If one method works better in some cases and another in others, their fields of operation nevertheless overlap in some places. Knowledge of different methods gives the doctor a greater range of therapies from which to choose the best in a particular case. He will thus be acting in the best interests of his patients by responding directly to their demands.

We have both practised homoeopathy for a number of years and have established that, though this method of treatment cannot be used to solve every single medical problem, it has been quite possible to use it in the majority of cases which we have met within a private practice.

Apart from the significant therapeutic techniques it offered, we found that it provided a different way of approaching the patient, another model for establishing diagnosis and applying treatment, which had two advantages: it gave a complete picture of individual patients, and it gave us the ability to determine, as soon as the patient consulted us, what should be given priority treatment, either with homoeopathic remedies or by other means.

This system—which, as we have said, was first conceived at the end of the 18th century—has been very largely obscured and excluded from the medical canon, finding itself consigned to the realms of fringe medicine. Yet Hahnemann, its founder, was the first doctor to demonstrate that serious study of any form of therapy demands systematic experimentation, and for this he gave the precise ground-rules. In the therapeutic jungle which existed at the time, he suggested a method of studying the pharmacological action of medicaments which had until then been used only empirically. He defined the rules for experiment and prescription and imposed a system of medical logic by codifying the method of examining the patient. He advised that the patient be considered as a special individual and, in the matter of prescription, that greatest weight should be given to those symptoms most characteristic of each person's particular reaction.

He was wrong, it seems, in his concept of 'vital force', and in thinking that illness was the consequence of a disturbance or imbalance in this vital force. Can we really mock him for that? Was there any alternative hypothesis to the idea of vitalism at that time? As François Jacob has said, there was no other means of understanding the process of life unless one opted for a purely mechanistic concept of Man as a machine, something which makes us smile even more today. There is little point in upbraiding a man who subscribed to some of the prevalent ideas of his age, especially since, in many other ways, he was very greatly ahead of his time. So let us concentrate instead objectively on the positive legacy he left us:

Firstly, an original method of observing the patient and of prescribing. Secondly, a new pharmacopoeia, giving a precise description of 114 clearly defined medicines. Thirdly, a precise technique of improving this pharmacopoeia: using this technique, his pupils and successors have studied the action of more than 2000 different substances of animal, mineral and, most often, vegetable origin. Fourthly, rules governing dosage, so that medicaments are administered in extremely weak, non-toxic doses.

All four teachings are based on a general biological law, the *law of similars*. Maybe Hahnemann was wrong to think that this law was always applicable; wrong to judge that his method was the only acceptable one, the only one able to govern medicine; wrong also to state his case so forcefully, thereby unleashing violent polemic as a reaction against him. But, here, as in so many other areas of medicine, everyone, homoeopath and allopath alike, forgets the facts and concentrates on the ideas, either hurling mutual opprobrium or simply terminating all communication on the subject. Too much time is wasted in sterile arguments of this type. It is much more worthwhile to present the facts as rigorously and objectively as possible—not in an attempt to win over the diehards of whatever belief or discipline, but rather to show those who are dissatisfied, who are questioning, that there is an alternative and remarkable method of treatment available to those who know how to administer it.

CHAPTER II

How I Became a Homoeopathic Doctor

In October 1952 I set up in practice in a little village in the Charente district. My medical career was beginning without any worries or major problems, just as I had hoped.

The house, a former rectory, was large and comfortable, in spite of its age and dilapidation. The village was a pleasant one, its inhabitants apparently satisfied and well disposed towards me. There had never been a doctor in the parish before, but I was shown a house where a medical officer had lived during the last century. There I discovered a strange 'sweating machine', a sort of wooden box in which my ingenious predecessor used to shut up his patient, surrounded by sacks of hot oats 'to bring out the badness'. Here, for the first time since the beginning of my medical work, I was confronted with a treatment based on general ideas very different from my own. However, such alternative ideas had yet to attract my attention. My interest was confined to the folk-lore aspect of the device, and it did not cross my mind that there could be more to it. In fact, my own ideas were based on a few simple principles: first and foremost I was a technician, so what had this nonsense to do with me? I was there to apply a technique, the one I had learnt and which, furthermore, suited me very well. Full stop: that was all.

Such a categorical declaration may seem strange, to say the least, now, in the 1980s, at a time when 'technical' medicine is being criticised and decried, if not totally rejected, by certain people (writers rather than doctors) who are more inclined to dream about reality than to live it.

I had begun my studies in 1945, just after the war, and qualified as a doctor in 1952. Considerable progress had just been made in medicine. Penicillin had arrived in France with the Americans and, with several other antibiotics, was beginning unchallenged its triumphant and cloudless reign. Thus I had the opportunity of using streptomycin right from its inception. I was at that time an extern dealing with infectious diseases, and my work consisted (among other things) of giving spinal injections of streptomycin every morning to patients suffering from tubercular meningitis. Most of these patients recovered, where previously they would all have died, a diagnosis of tubercular meningitis being the equivalent of a death sentence. Some simple technical rules, based on clinical examination and the prescription of chemotherapy, made it possible to save the lives of patients who, like many others, had up to then been unconditionally condemned to death. So I was glad to be just a technician, and questioned nothing.

Good fortune in the competitive examinations had made it possible for me to become an extern at the end of my first year in medicine, and two years later to be made a provisional intern. I lived-in at the Tondu hospital and attended the medical school only for certain important lectures and to take my written examinations. At that time the life of a medical student was divided into two parts: theorectical study at the school of medicine, and practical work at the hospital. There was an examination each year at the medical school which counted towards one's medical doctorate, and a competitive examination at the hospital for the posts of extern and intern.

I had already made my choice: I preferred practice to theory. Life at the hospital, divided between the daily supervision of in-patients and spells of duty in the casualty wards, took up the greater part of my time. I was learning the responses which defined the limits of my activities, becoming progressively more aware of what I could do, how I could do it, and when it was necessary for me to refer to someone else—and, if so, to whom.

These responses, simple as they may appear, are of very great importance, since they enable every doctor to be aware at the same time both of his possibilities and of his limitations. They, and they alone, form the kernel of all medical activity, at whatever level it may be. They are the indispensable bulwark of all medical practice. I shall have occasion to refer to this again several times, since this major rule is all too often forgotten by those who glorify in 'practising alternative medicine'.

This hospital life had a slightly artificial character; but I did not realise this until much later, long after I had set up in practice. Without indulging in caricature or facile criticism, we must recognise, whether we like it or not, that in those days we paid little attention to our patients as people, even if after several weeks they were no longer complete strangers to us. It is true that we had information about their lives, their family circumstances and their jobs; but this knowledge had only an anecdotal interest for us. They were primarily sick people— that is to say, individuals suffering from an illness—and their illness was all that interested us. This was what we wanted to study or, more precisely, to isolate as far as possible from its context. We therefore systematically researched the objective, measurable and quantifiable symptoms, and listened with only half an ear to the *subjective* symptoms through which the patient's true complaint was expressed.

Thus, little by little, a system was built up in my mind which delimited my courses of action in establishing relation-ships and bringing or not bringing to light this or that symptom. This framework, although undeniably interesting, useful and efficacious, was nonetheless compartmentalised and restrictive. It is certainly not my intention to seek its destruc-tion or even its devaluation: all I wish to do is to point out that there exist other systems with other terms of reference, which may give significance to symptoms which have hitherto been overlooked or regarded as valueless. Whatever one may say, these systems are not necessarily opposed or contradictory. They can complement one another, thus opening up a broader field of action to medical practice, rather than restricting it by fixing arbitrary limits.

As I say, the system worked and still does work very well,

both in the hospital context and outside it. I was able to see this for myself when acting as locum at Bordeaux, where I worked one day a week with a colleague, and in the country during the summer holidays. I conscientiously applied the rules I had learnt: examination, diagnosis, treatment. I did, however, notice one difference from the hospital: the diagnoses were more often simple ones, easy to make without complicated examinations. As for the therapy, it consisted solely in prescribing a few medicines which, at least in the short term, were effective and rapid.

A new realisation dawned on me. Among my daily consultations there were few really 'sick' people; that is to say, people suffering from a characteristic illness. Most complained of troubles which had no significance. A few kind words and the prescription of a few soothing medicines for the circulation, the digestion or the nerves were all that were needed for my peace of mind. On the one hand, then, there were the 'true sick', those suffering from an illness which I could diagnose or which, if necessary, I could arrange to have investigated at the hospital; on the other hand, there were the 'false sick', those who complained of feeling ill but in whom I was unable to find anything which I had learnt about. In such cases the little red prescription handbook, which I kept by me all the time, was a valuable and reassuring aid.

Armed with these few possessions, I set up in practice and confidently began my professional career.

I had the feeling of being a technician well trained by the medical establishment, and I felt myself capable of applying its rules. My rôle seemed to me to be a simple one: I had to investigate the malady as I had been taught, determine what it was, isolate it and treat it, either with the medical means within my own scope or by surgery. This function as front-line soldier consisted also of recognising certain symptoms, the ones I had been taught were significant, and in using them to make a diagnosis and decide on therapy. If I was not always capable of making an exact diagnosis, I could at least find out and recognise what was going to need urgent treatment and what, on the other hand, could wait. I was the first link in the medical chain and, if in the slightest doubt, I would send my patient either to the clinic or to the hospital in the neighbouring town, where diagnosis could be made or confirmed and, at the same time, technical treatment carried out.

Everything was in order. The hierarchy was perfect, everyone having their appointed place, just as in the hospital when I had been a student. I felt secure. The system suited me and gave me complete satisfaction, particularly in the two fields which were, at the start, my chief areas of activity, surgical pathology and the use of antibiotics.

Equipped to carry out minor surgery, I incised abscesses, and took my own X-rays, which I developed in a little darkroom underneath the stairs. I set fractures, I sewed up accident cases, I extracted foreign bodies where possible. All this was done in the consulting-room itself, with very simple means which would make many young doctors smile nowadays, but which were nevertheless effective. As I have said, for more serious operations I would send my patient to the hospital or the private clinic, but for an urgent case—appendicitis, extra-uterine swelling, open fracture, or loss of a limb in an accident, for example—I would put him in my car and drive him there myself. The surgeon was there: the patient was examined and the operation performed, often with my assistance. Once again, I was integrated into a medical team.

These trips were an opportunity for me to meet other colleagues from my area who had, like myself, accompanied their patients or who were present at operations. I took advantage of these chance meetings to chat, to obtain news about various people and to learn about medical matters, such as epidemics and mutual problems.

The surgical clinic was an excellent meeting-place. Medical life went on there with a rhythm and according to rites which were familiar to me: I had known similar ones when a student at the hospital. Here, too, the system continued to function in a perfectly coherent manner. However, in conversation with colleagues older than myself who had been in practice longer, I noticed a sort of lassitude, of disillusion, which surprised me all the more because I did not understand it. My own interest in my chosen profession remained as lively as ever.

Practical work on the spot—that is to say, in the patients' own homes—also continued to give me satisfaction. I was called in only for serious and acute cases, mostly those with a history of infection. It might be a violent sore throat, which kept the patient in bed with a temperature of 40°C (104°F) and serious loss of appetite. Antibiotics were prescribed, a urine-analysis requested. Sometimes it would be a more persistent sore throat, where the patient was more exhausted, his throat in a bad state with white spots or greyish patches, and with painful swellings in the neck. A swab would be taken and sent to the laboratory; a course of antibiotics would be started but the possibility of serum therapy had also to be considered, because cases of diphtheria were still being reported. Other times it would be an acute attack of bronchitis, pleuritis or pleurisy, sometimes cystitis or a boil; but on occasion the case was far more serious.

I remember the 'phone ringing at about six o'clock one evening. 'He has a sore throat, a headache and a temperature,' I was told; he lived on the Angoulême road. As I was not too busy, I decided to dine early and call at his house on my way to the cinema, where I had arranged to take my wife. I stopped my car in the yard and found my patient in bed. His temperature was 40°C (104°F), and he complained of a violent headache and pains in his muscles. He could not move and had just vomited. A quick examination revealed stiffness at the nape of the neck and difficulty in sitting up. I immediately diagnosed an attack of meningitis. I took out a sterile test-tube and a needle, and made the patient crouch like a gun-dog. With my wife's help, I performed a lumbar puncture: the liquid was cloudy. Without further ado, I had the patient dressed, put him in my car, and drove to Angoulême to the hospital—not to the cinema as we had arranged! Cerebrospinal meningitis was confirmed. Fortunately everything turned out well.

Part of my work consisted of attending confinements. At that time these took place at home since, in the minds of the pregnant women and their families, the clinic was only for difficult deliveries. This meant that some of the home births took place in strange conditions, both as regards the confinement itself and as regards the simple rules of hygiene. All this went on under the approving or disapproving eyes of neighbours who considered themselves experienced in such matters, and who were all uncompromising partisans in favour of myself or one or other of my colleagues. It was a real relief to me after I had helped to set up public clinics where I could take my patients, personally supervise them and deliver the babies in favourable conditions, backed up by an experienced team.

At that time the field of antibiotics gave every assurance of of success. Indeed, it was the ideal specialisation for a satisfying and rewarding medical practice, thanks to the simplicity of the process involved. An organism—by definition, in good health—meets a microbe, and illness develops. A therapy, based on the aetiology of the condition, is introduced. An antibiotic is prescribed, the microbe is killed and the patient is restored to health. It is true that infectious diseases take different forms according to different microbes; but the microbes had not yet become resistant, the number of antibiotics available on the market was smaller, and the practical results were excellent.

Satisfactory as this therapy was, it soon became wearisome as a result of its systematic repetition. Aided by habit, one's clinical judgement, instead of developing, ends up by becoming blunted. As for one's responses, they may become quicker and more effective in certain ways, but most often they lose their accuracy. Thus some very typical symptoms are investigated systematically, while other more minor ones are purposely ignored. The result is that the everyday treatment of symptoms becomes even simpler and more routine. Certainly this process, which is being adopted increasingly, does have some advantages—emergency surgical or medical therapy can be carried out quickly and acute conditions can the better be treated—but it is not without its disadvantages: the scope of research becomes more and more restricted, and the doctor remains in total ignorance of another kind of pathology, a type not included in his training.

Little by little I was to come to know this other pathology. Obviously I was not and, in my village, could not be a specialist of whatever competence in infectious diseases, nor could I pick and choose my kind of specialisation, for the patients who came to see me, or who asked me to visit them at home, presented all sorts of very different problems. They did not necessarily fit into the simple categories which constituted the whole of my medical knowledge at that time. It was not always easy for me to make a definite diagnosis, to discover the cause of the disease and to prescribe treatment. I did what I had been taught to do—and, indeed, I still think it is absolutely necessary to carry out this procedure every time a doctor is faced with a new patient: he must try to find out what is wrong, make a clear diagnosis, and prescribe a logical therapy, at the same time bearing in mind that this is not always feasible. Most patients do not have 'copybook' maladies, so that an exact diagnosis may be impossible and the treatment, which the doctor has in each case to improvise, apt to be somewhat arbitrary.

It is a great temptation to classify patients as (a) those suffering from a specific illness and (b) those suffering from a functional complaint. Such a precise distinction not only is simplistic but also relieves the doctor of responsibility: as we have seen there are the 'true patients', who are worthy of attention, the 'false patients', who believvve themselves to be ill, but are not, according to the terms of reference which themedical profession has itself chosen. In both cases there is no need to worry. To the first category you apply the strict technical rules; to the second, as soon as they have been duly recognised as such, you say a few kind words and prescribe some medicines, which you know perfectly well are ineffective placebos.

This strict classification system is only of short-term value. It can be accepted by a doctor who sees his patients for only a short space of time, during a brief stay in hospital or when the doctor is acting as a locum (which generally lasts for not more than a month), or when he is setting up in practice.

After several years in practice, however, the real questions arise: Are the criteria which I have been given, which I have had impressed upon me and which I have accepted, really the only valid ones? If an illness must be investigated, is it natural to discount and pass over all complaints except the actual malady? If the objective signs alone are 'reliable', do the subjective symptoms really have no value at all? Could they not be regarded as indicative signs which can help you to determine what is going on and foresee what may be about to develop?

The leaving of all these questions in abeyance, unanswered, made me dissatisfied, and I became better able to understand the disillusion which tinged the conversations of my colleagues and the feeling they had of being reduced to the status of a sort of robot with semi-automatic movements, a machine for dispensing medicines. I was able to sympathise with the kind of rebellion which made them make a stand against the ever-increasing control by the state, the social-security services and the drug houses which produced the medicines. I became aware of their feeling of helplessness in the face of the progressive diminishment of their prerogatives in favour of specialists entrenched behind ever more powerful and more costly equipment. I sensed their ill-humour towards patients who were becoming progressively more peremptory and more demanding. It is true that this attitude was scarcely perceptible in the country, where the people were more traditionalist, less receptive to technical advances and also more suspicious of any kind of excess. However, even if my limited and faithful patients did not openly express dissatisfaction, they still made me reflect about work: 'I provide a technical solution for the problems with which I am faced: this part of my rôle is fulfilled completely. But it is clear that not all problems can be solved in this way. Even if they can be solved temporarily, subsequent relapses show clearly that, behind the apparent state of improvement, something else is taking place, which for the moment is beyond my comprehension.'

I was getting to know my patients better and better. I saw them living their daily lives, I met them often, and I realised that, between physical injuries or functional diseases with a precise mechanism on the one hand, and psychiatric disorders on the other, there existed a territory occupied by various troubles which did not fit into any category. At that time the idea of psychosomatic illness had not yet been born—or, at least, not to a country doctor: there was some talk of it, it is true, and you read a few articles about it, but that was as far as your knowledge of such marginal things went. Still, I felt that I must do something, but I did not know what.

As a family doctor, in the true sense of the term, I treated whole families: children, parents, grandparents and often aunts and uncles. More often than not, they all lived in one community on the same farm or on neighbouring farms. The bond of trust between doctor and patients was very great, and I would know that so-and-so, who had had a nerve displaced, had seen the bone-setter, or that Louise had had distant healing based on a photograph from a healer in Deux-Sèvres for her attacks of nerves: 'It is quite natural, you know, when orthodox medicine cannot do anything for them.' From the neighbours I learnt, too, that when Marcel had had pleurisy his wife had taken an unwashed shirt to old Matthieu in the next village and he had confirmed my diagnosis: 'That's just as good as an X-ray and, besides, two opinions are better than one.' These tales amused me all the more because Matthieu was one of my staunchest patients: he might have been perfectly competent to detect illness in others, but he could not identify it in his own case, and preferred to consult the doctor!

From time to time, when I was visiting a case of measles or someone who had been injured at work, I would ask after other members of the family. In one, not a typical, case it was the grandfather: 'How is he? How is his bronchitis? I haven't seen him this winter. Has he gone to live with his daughter at Cognac?' 'No, he is still here, but he is quite well. He hardly ever has a cold nowadays. It has all passed off. He looks after the animals. His resistance is better than it used to be.'

This intrigued me. I knew the old man well—a bronchitic old fellow with sclerotic lungs. He often used to send for me in the winter when he had a bad attack, which would respond well to antibiotics but then would easily relapse again. What had happened? They admitted timidly, with digressions and pauses so as not to offend me: 'Some friends told him to go in for homoeopathy. He didn't do it at once. He didn't want to, you know, because he had faith in you; but in the end ... he let himself be persuaded, and he went. Since then he has not regretted it. He is much better. You should have a chat about it one day.'

I had never heard any talk about homoeopathy, either for or against it, except for occasional allusions to our colleague in Angoulême—not very favourable ones, it is true, but not spiteful either.

I came across other patients who had been treated in the same way: asthmatics, rheumatics, those who said they were suffering from functional complaints. Some of them showed me little white pills in a glass tube with nothing on the label but a Latin word followed by a number: Sulphur 7c, Thuya 9c. In my mind I rather summarily put homoeopaths in the same category as faith-healers and thought: 'So much the better for the patient. After all, there wasn't much wrong with him. He believes in the treatment and it makes him feel better—that's good. But we shall see what happens if he, is ever *really* ill.'

I did not lose any sleep over the matter: my curiosity had yet to be awakened and my pride was hardly touched. My territory had not yet been invaded; in fact, I didn't feel it fell within my purlieu at all, for in my eyes it did not count as medicine at all.

As time went on, however, the number of my patients cured by homoeopathy increased and I had a strange feeling. Although I did not recognise many of them as being ill, according to my criteria, there were others who really *were* ill. Chronic bronchitics, for example, whom I had known for years and who had been classed as such after X-rays and examination of their sputum, and whom I had had to put on antibiotics all winter. Rheumatics, too, suffering from chronic arthritis, whose X-rays I kept and whom I had often seen laid up. There was even a woman suffering from progressive chronic poly-arthritis who, although not cured, was now living comfortably without needing any major anti-inflammation treatment and with the rate of crystal-formation in her synovial fluid. There were former eczematics for whom ointments and various coloured solutions had done nothing except to bring slight, temporary relief; and migraine sufferers, asthmatics ...

It was at this point that I decided to go to see this homoeopath

He was a charming man and gave me a very friendly reception. We chatted about my patients, especially about the ones he had seen. I gave him several names. He brought out some files on which he had noted his observations and the medicines he had prescribed; then other files on patients which we did not share, with notes and letters. He explained his procedure to me, how he studied his patients and how he determined his prescriptions, and he told me about his concept of illness. It was all new to me: a new method with very precise rules for observing the patient, an unaccustomed therapy, a special concept of illness.

My colleague was a serious man. His conversation was free from self-aggrandisement and his obsersations were clear. There was no doubt that his patients were well examined and well studied, and that a diagnosis was made wherever possible. The method of prescription was logical. I noticed, too, that some patients were treated not by homoeopathy but by more orthodox techniques. In this way he showed me the limitations and the scope of his therapy. I had no reason to doubt his words, his seriousness or his modesty.

I went away astonished, taking several books with me. My convictions were somewhat shaken. Technical medicine existed and it worked. It was based on known laws, as my colleague himself agreed. But parallel with it there existed other thereapeutic methods applicable to the large number of patients for whom I was reduced to improvising; and above all there was one method which apprently made it possible to understand the ailments and to treat them in a clear and logical manner. I discovered that, without abandoning my own therapies, it was possible for me to widen the scope of my knowledge, to go a little further.

I set about reading the books I had taken home. What a

surprise and what a disappointment! While my colleague's talk had been based on precise facts, these books contained a mixture of correct observations and unlikely stories. An apparently impeccable rationality in the observation of facts was allied quite unashamedly with total irrationality on the level of explanation and theory. There was talk of constitutions, of miasmas, of toxins, of drainages, of inherited and acquired characteristics and of astrological types, plus references to long-abandoned theories. All this was stated and expounded with a complacence and a lack of restraint which really shocked me.

Far be it from me, I thought, to wish to reject the teaching of the medical school, whose real value I knew, in order to subscribe unconditionally to the dogma underlying these writings! There was no question of my abandoning the orthodox therapy which I knew was, at least in certain fields, effective.

In disappointment I refrained from treating my chronic patients while at the same time trying to look at them in a different way. I questioned them and realised that, unknown to me, many had indeed been treated by homoeopathy. It was impossible for me to deny a certain number of positive results. I asked to see their presescriptions to find out which medicines had been used. I read up the *materia medica* concerning these medicines, and I learnt their properties, their clinical indications and the correct way of prescribing them.

Not only did I rediscover the rational approach I was seeking, at the same time there came back to me the words of my friend about his technique, his way of choosing the medicine best adapted to the patient who was consulting him. I remembered, too, that he had not delved into any explanatory theory, but had been content to help me envisage illness as a simple disorder taking different forms in different individuals, always stressing that some were more susceptible than others to this or that illness. He had told me that behind each illness there was a 'constitutional background' which was favourable to its development, and that knowledge of this background made it possible for one to anticipate and ward off serious troubles. This notion I welcomed eagerly. I had already been told about the constitutional background in the course of my studies and it was discussed in all the books; but never before had there been any question of acting on it in any way, and so its status had remained little higher than that of a myth. The homoeopathic concept of the background, on the other hand, appeared to me to be operational.

I went to see my colleague again. I saw some more of his notes. I came to understand the method better—and I decided, on his advice, not to worry about the theory but to experiment with certain medicines in certain specific cases, notably of whooping-cough, where, according to him, five or six medicines could be useful, the three chief ones being *Drosera*, *Belladonna* and *Coccus cacti*. He showed me how to choose and how to prescribe them.

I had, up to then, been very worried about the children with whooping-cough. It is a common illness and, although less serious after the age of two, it nevertheless remains exhausting both for the child and for the family. It can drag on for months, and the doctor is almost powerless to do anything about it apart from having given preventative vaccination in the first place. Cough-syrups, suppositories and advising the patient to take a change of air or even a trip in an aeroplane were the only means we had then to stop the incessant fits of coughing. As everyone knows, whooping-cough is not psychosomatic, but is an infectious disease caused by Bordet-Gengou's bacillus, which is characterised by paroxysms of the distinctive coughing. These much dreaded fits are often accompanied by the bringing up of long strands of phlegm, and are frequently followed by vomiting. Unable to destroy the microbe responsible, we were reduced to using medicines chosen completely at random in an attempt to alleviate the symptoms. The parents of the sufferers often gave old wives' remedies, such as, for example, the slime of a snail, chosen on the principle of analogy—this substance resembles the strands of phlegm coughed up by the child. As I was to learn later, this practice was a relic of the doctrine of signatures, often confused with homoeopathy.

I had definitely noticed that, even though the whooping-cough patients had several symptoms in common which made the disease easy to diagnose, the illness did not take the same course in all of them, and that the clinical expression of the illness contained aspects which differed from subject to subject; but these observations had not been of any use to me in prescribing my treatment. If I wanted to use homoeopathic medicine, on the other hand, I must study carefully the symptoms of each sufferer before prescribing.

One child would turn purple during his coughing-fits; another would be pale and covered with sweat; one would be disturbed and cry before coughing; another would stop playing and wait quietly for the fit to come on. All these symptoms, which had been totally irrelevant to me up to now, become indispensable in choosing the right homoeopathic prescription.

Shortly after my visit to Angoulême, my own three children had whooping-cough. I immediately tried out on them the remedies advised by my colleague, noting their particular reactions. Surprisingly, this attack of whooping-cough was mild; it disappeared quickly and completely. I did not initially attach any great importance to this as not all attacks of whooping-cough are serious.

The episode took place during a whooping-cough epidemic: a number of children in the village and in neighbouring villages caught it. I was able to put to the test the various homoeopathic medicines which had been suggested to me. I obtained a totally unexpected result: the attacks very quickly cured, so quickly that I wondered if they had been real ones. However, this outcome was repeated again and again, and I noted a surprising fact. In the villages where there were two or three of the doctors at work, it was only in the children whom I treated that the illness took a mild form. I had to accept the evidence: homoeopathic medicines were very effective. I was also surprised to learn how cheap they were and, therefore, that the cost of the whole treatment was in no way comparable with the cost of orthodox treatment.

My patients were so pleased with this therapy that they advised their neighbours to buy the same medicines. Some profited by this advice and obtained good results; others, on the contrary, benefited from it not at all. This proved that homoeopathy did not consist of an omnibus treatment given merely on the basis of the name of the illness and its diagnosis. As my colleague had explained to me, the prescription could not be effective unless it was drawn up with respect to the particular reaction of the patient. I had, therefore, to observe my patients more closely than I had done in the past.

Suddenly I saw my career from a different angle, and my work took on a new interest. The straightforward diagnosis 'whooping-cough'—so typical, quick and easy—became a more rewarding exercise; the bouts of epidemic no longer seemed to me so tiring as they had been before. Indeed, for some time I had been feeling that I was becoming involved in a mere chain of work: sore throat = antibiotics, bronchitis = antibiotics, stomach ulcer = bismuth, and so on. What had my function been reduced to? Instead of studying the patient by listening to him and trying to understand him, I had been concentrating entirely on the disease. I was deliberately restricting the scope of my investigations so as to look at only those symptoms upon which I could base my diagnosis, and making my prescriptions using only a few medicines—albeit extremely effective ones. But such prescription, stemming from my ever more reduced field of observation, took on a stereotyped form, which was misleading in the long run.

Since having decided to treat my patients by homoeopathy, I saw them in a new light. I observed them differently although without in any way abandoning my existing technique. I had simply extended my repertoire.

There arose in my mind a curious impression, simultaneously both pleasant and unpleasant, as I progressed along these lines. The pleasure of discovery was mixed with a feeling of frustration, even to the extent that I felt I had been morally swindled. Why had I been taught to research only certain symptoms, to find significance in them at the expense of others which were equally interesting and equally significant? Why had I never been told about the latter? To what end had they been suppressed? Why had the scope of medicine been

45

voluntarily limited to a single one of its aspects, however important that aspect might be?

In homoeopathy I had suddenly discovered another aspect of medicine: another means of investigation, understanding and action had now been suggested to me. I discussed it with my colleagues; there was a general burst of laughter. It was completely ridiculous. I had gone mad. Everyone 'knew' that those medicines were no use. The patients recovered of their own accord. They were only 'false patients', 'neurotics', 'cranks' ready to believe any kind of nonsense. 'Come on, old chap, be reasonable. Keep your feet on the ground,' they told me. There was no logic, no reasoning in their remarks: to my mind, all their arguments were emotional; none of them were convincing. The reaction was purely and simply a refusal to observe certain facts objectively, and to reconsider medical practice and teaching; coupled with the no less energetic refusal to become involved oneself. I found around me not only incomprehension but, above all, a positive desire not to see, not to know, not to experiment, not to make life more complicated.

In spite of this, everyone recognised and appreciated the moral and professional honesty of my homoeopathic colleague and also his ability as a doctor; but that did not stop them from declaring with a knowing smile that he only treated 'false patients'. This was not at all my opinion. I had seen results with 'true patients', in the orthodox meaning of the term, and it would have needed very bad faith indeed to declare after the event—or, rather, after a cure—that I had been mistaken, that the diagnosis had been wrong. To my mind, such an attitude would have been the height of dishonesty.

Despite their sarcasm, I decided to go on studying homoeopathy and to treat certain of my patients by it. I chose simple, clear cases; the results I obtained were all the more interesting because they depended entirely on the precision and the limit of my observations and examinations. I no longer had, as formerly, the reassuring protection of antibiotics—although I kept the latter in reserve for cases where improvement was too slow in appearing, since I was not yet quite certain of the effects of medicines which were so new to me.

I had the satisfaction of often seeing my acute patients recover very quickly, with an extremely short period of convalescence—much shorter than I had been used to observing previously. These results gave me confidence and encouraged me to go on.

I came more and more to treat homoeopathically the chronically sick, those suffering from functional ailments, and the so-called 'false sick'—those who, quite simply, did not fit into the medical system because they did not correspond to its norms. I realised that these represented 70% to 80% of my patients.

For those patients not recognisably sick, I had up to then been unable to do anything. I had been unprepared and powerless, and this lack of a suitable therapy incurred the risk either of throwing them into the arms of a faith-healer or of making them undergo excessive medication. On the one hand they would be escaping regular medical supervision, on the other they might be unnecessarily 'overprocessed', a fashionable term frightening in the dehumanisation it suggested.

In either case, there was danger for them, although not the same kind of danger. Between therapeutic abstention and medicinal abuse, between leaving them to the tender mercies of nature and risking overmedication, I was becoming aware of the existence of another way. Its practice required of me a quite different kind of attention, a quite different way of listening—every consultation would take me at least half an hour. Indeed, in addition to the ordinary examination and interrogation common to all doctors, I had to conduct a detailed grilling which revealed to me the personal reactivity of each patient, so that I could choose the medicine or medicines best suited to his particular case: if in cases of acute illness the therapy to be prescribed is quick and easy, it is not the same in cases of chronic illness.

With an acute illness, once the diagnosis has been made, the choice is reduced to four or five possible medicines. A few precise questions are sufficient to determine the remedy. With influenza, for example, the particular symptoms of congestion of the head, muscular curvature, a general sensation of numbness or even coarseness would make you choose *Gelse-mium*. On the other hand, the symptoms of pains in the bones, pains in the frontal region and the sinuses, and pains in the eyeballs aggravated by the simple movement of the eyes would make you advise *Eupatorium perfoliatum*. The action of these remedies, chosen at random from among others, is extremely quick if they are strongly indicated. A curious fact for me, at least at the beginning of my practice of homoeopathy, was that I noticed that the period of convalescence was practically non existent. As soon as the patient was cured, he felt in excellent form and ready to go back to work.

Winter brought its toll of infectious diseases, colds, bronchitis and influenza. The adults were often reluctant to accept a homoeopathic prescription: most were still under the spell of antibiotics—they asked for them and were disappointed if I refused to grant their request. On the other hand, this therapy was much better received on behalf of children and by the children themselves. No more jabs, no more suppositories, no more syrups or medicines with a possibly stomach-wrenching taste, which one usually had to adminster by force in the midst of tears and screams. There was none of that; just some little sweets, some little round, white balls to suck every two or three hours. It was much easier for the parents, much nicer for the children. People accepted the change as much in order not to upset the youngsters as to please me, the doctor.

Ear inflammations were legion. They might be severe or insidious, as for example a long drawn-out bout of nasopharyngitis, and were generally treated at that time by antibiotics, which often necessitated a course being administered at home, for the young children or, for the older ones, at the clinic in town. Yet I found a few homoeopathic remedies were sufficient. I used to see pallid children, who had been suffering from a cold for several days, crying quietly and holding their ears. Their temperature would be round about 38° or 38.5°C, (100.4 or 101.3°F) the throat and the nasopharynx slightly inflamed, and one or both tympana congested. One or two doses of *Pyrogenium* and a few granules of *Ferrum phosphoricum* sucked every two hours would put everything right again, to the great satisfaction of all concerned: the parents whose worries were put at rest; the child, who did not have to be given an injection; and the doctor, who was surprised that he had not known about these medicines earlier!

Sometimes I was rung up at night. A little girl had woken up screaming. Her temperature was high. I had to get up, dress and go to see her. 'Is it serious, doctor? It came on all of a sudden; she was asleep. We had just gone to bed. She was all right yesterday: she was playing in the yard all evening. There was a lot of wind, true. Her grandmother did say to us: "You don't look after her. Poor little thing, she'll get pleurisy". Or perhaps it's her teeth. What do you think, doctor?'

The little girl was ill, that was obvious. She was restless and burning hot. Her temperature was 40°C, (104°F), her abdomen was supple, there was no painful place on it, no diarrhoea, no vomiting, the nape of her neck was easily moved, there were no unusual sounds in her chest, her throat was quite normal, but the left tympanum was very red. *Aconite* was prescribed: two or three doses at ten minute intervals, then once or twice during the night if the child awoke. A clinical check was made the next day for safety's sake. All was well: the symptoms had disappeared.

At other times there might be a feverish, exhausted child, sweating profusely, her hair damp with perspiration and with a brilliantly red throat with enormous tonsils. A few pillules of *Belladonna* and *Mercurius* alternately every hour, and in forty-eight hours it had all passed.

These problems were simple ones, easily solved. Every day I learnt that, in addition to the objective symptoms (aspects of the throat and the tympanum), the discovery of certain others was equally valuable during a feverish attack in determing the choice of a homoeopathic remedy—the presence or absence of perspiration, for example, nervous agitation or depression, and many other signs.

In the case of chronic illness the problems were far more complicated, it is true, but at the same time far more interesting. It was already a great satisfaction to be able to treat sore throats, bronchitis and inflammations of the ear with medicines which were easy to use, cost little and were not toxic. Besides, I never saw any secondary effects, as I did when antibiotics had been administered—tiredness, digestive troubles, inflammation of the tongue, mycosis or various allergic reactions. These were minor troubles, usually of short duration and easily acceptable when an extremely serious infection justified the taking of antibiotics, but they were infuriating when such a prescription was not urgently needed, and had had to be applied only for want of something better. Faced with common and repeated infections, what else could we suggest but antibiotics? We had nothing else at our disposal, we had no other solution.

However, choosing homoeopathic therapy—new as it was to me—did not entirely solve the problem: the sore throats and earaches were cured, but still they recurred again. It was necessary for me to understand what governed the appearance of these repeated infections, and to do this I had to study the patients as distinct from their severe attacks, and thus go one step further and learn to use the so-called 'constitutional remedies' of homoeopathy, the medicines which were able to modify in depth the reactivity of the patient—that is to say, his or her particular susceptibility to this or that illness.

Some of the elements involved I had hitherto overlooked: the morphology of the patient, his general comportment, his character, his way of living, his individual reaction to heat or cold and to difficulties, whether he reacted with anger or submission, and his activity or passivity, as well as the various illnesses he had had, the way he had had them, the chief circumstances in his life which could have influenced his behaviour, the family sphere in which he lived and many other things as well. It meant that I had to listen to the patient, watch him living, understand him and try to establish his capacity for adaptation, to define the limits within which he could lead a life in equilibrium, the equilibrium being his own particular one.

All this was extremely interesting, but it meant that I had to have a considerable amount of time at my disposal, and it required from the patient a great deal of participation for which he was not prepared and the novelty of which for the most part surprised him. For him, as for me, it was not always possible. On the one hand there was my life as a country doctor, a constant rush between visits, consultations, urgent summonses to accidents and confinements; on the other there was the patient, coming to ask for immediate relief from his passing indisposition and entirely preoccupied by it—and, over-awed by the apparent omnipotence of medical science, requesting, or even sometimes demanding, a quick solution to the problem which was worrying him at that moment. Medicine was able to relieve him and it was its duty to do so instantly and, if possible, for nothing; he was paying quite enough for it and it was his right! The newest, the most effective and the most expensive medicines were what he wanted ... until the next time.

Nowadays there tend to be fewer patients of this kind; in fact, the assumed omnipotence of medicine has taken a battering for a variety of reasons, some of them surprising. The new wave of 'ecology', to which everyone refers (though each in his own way), is carrying all before it, bringing to our consulting rooms a new kind of patient looking for 'natural' remedies, 'harmless' herbs, and, more or less original diets —if not to say eccentric ones—and fiercely refusing antibiotics and vaccinations. Beneath an apparently sane and innocuous outward appearance, this infatuation, this sudden taste for 'nature' hides a very real danger—as is inevitable when people abandon their 'common sense' and, in the name of blind faith in a particular doctirine which suits their personal taste, will stomach anything provided it is 'natural'. Such people are ready to inadvertently let their children die of tetanus or cerebrospinal meningitis.

My interest, then, in studying the patient in his totality grew to the same extent that the interest I had previously taken in the disease itself diminished. I am not saying that the importance assigned to a disease in isolation, to the analysis of diseases, should disappear, but my curiosity for this kind of study lessened. I wanted to practise in a different way; but this new kind of practice required a great deal of time. Indeed, it was becoming very difficult to respond to the urgent calls which are the customary lot of a country doctor, and at the same time to give all those new patients long consultatons which required my complete attention.

I therefore decided to set up in practice in Angoulême and to consult only by appointment. In this way my consultations took on a very different nature. The patients whom I saw were coming to consult a *homoeopathic* doctor, and so were already prepared for a certain attitude, a certain therapeutic relationship. This fact needs to be pointed out, since the alteration of the doctor-patient relationship may in certain cases have a positive effect and in others a negative one.

The effect is positive when the patient knows that the doctor he has chosen to consult is prepared to examine him patiently and carefully and to listen to him attentively for a long time because he wants to understand him better. Here, as he has always wanted, the patient is being treated like a sick person and no longer like an ordinary, anonymous sufferer from a disease to which he cannot relate and which he cannot understand.

But the effect is negative if the patient comes with his head stuffed with more or less vague theories about homoeopathic medicine. He has read some books or some articles on the subject and has formed a false picture of it. He has come to see a magician—which I can never be—and his surprise at not seeing me wield a pendulum or practise the laying-on of hands is a genuine one. Often he is even astonished that I put so many questions, that I ask him to explain to me in what way he feels ill, and he resents this. After all, I really ought to *know*! To him I am a healer invested with arcane powers through the knowledge of a mysterious science and, what is more, a healer who is also a doctor; the title 'doctor' is both a guarantee and a token of a pact made with the devil, representing all the negative side of medicine. His only consolation is that he can get back the cost of the medicines I prescribe for him—the medicines only, for my consultation fee is not refundable since I am not part of the French National Health Service.

This is a problem which I would like to tackle, all the more so because it is never faced openly but only through innuendoes or cutting and peremptory assertions, which are in no way rational or objective responses. 'The doctors outside the Health Service want to be freed of fixed salaries in order to make a fortune. It's as simple as that!' 'They fix their fees according to their patients, or rather according to their patients' means'. 'Of course, they only take patients with fat wallets.' 'They don't declare their fees and don't pay tax.' 'They go in for class medicine, abandoning the really sick people without much money and devoting themselves to those who are not really sick and are ready to pay any price they charge.' They are all hasty judgements, summary opinions, showing better than anything else a general misunderstanding of the question.

However, for a homoeopathic doctor like myself, receiving fifteen to twenty patients a day, I see no choice at the moment but to remain outside the conventional system. Unfortunately, it is the patients who suffer. Because of the authorities, arbitrary decision, the amount refunded for their consultation is derisory. If they are surprised by this at first, they quickly realise that homoeopathic treatment is not expensive. Not only are the consultations spaced out at long intervals, every two or three months, but the homoeopathic medicines are modestly priced: the cost of a prescription will be about £5.00 for two months' treatment. Furthermore, since their general equilibrium has been restored, their resistance is increased: the number of minor indispositions is decreased and those they do incur can most often be treated by simple advice on self-medication.

As I said before, the patients who came to see me after my change in status were different from the ones I had been accustomed to treat before. It seems to me important to state precisely why this was so, in order not to start sterile and useless arguments between homoeopaths and non-homoeopaths, or even between doctors practising different specialities, or the same speciality but under different conditions—in hospital or in private practice, in town or in the country.

Patients choose their doctor according to a certain number of criteria, which we have already mentioned. Whatever one may say, the various disciplines are not interchangeable, even though that is the avowed or secret hope of the medical authorities, the bureaucrats, and various economists and associations which all try progressively to establish a standardisation of medical treatment. This could be done, strictly speaking, if only a purely technical treatment were carried out; but we know that for 80% of patients something totally different is needed, even if this 'something' is happening unknown to the patient and the doctor.

Each doctor has his own set of patients and can therefore give evidence only from personal experience. It would be wrong to try to draw general conclusions from this, or to claim general truths, which out of context would no longer appear so obvious. I know, for example, that I have cured a certain number of asthmatics, and I have sufficient evidence to justify this claim. I know, too, that patients who, I believe, and who, according to their neighbours or family, have been cured through my care, after a few consultations, did not come back to see me, but went elsewhere for treatment, without telling anyone. I know, too, that certain patients lied to me and took other medicines besides the ones I prescribed, going from theophylline to cortisone, but preferring to keep silent about such details.

The physician in private practice, whoever he may be, must remain clear and very critical about the apparent results he obtains, and must refrain from crowing over his successes—a tendency incompatible with the practice of medicine, especially when he is defending one method against another. Medical progress must not be grounded on passionate or partisan claims which obscure the real argument.

I can, therefore, report only what I have seen or what I thought I saw when applying the homoeopathic method. I hope in this way to show that alongside the favourite field of action of technical medicine—which I in no way seek to belittle—there exists 'something else' which deserves to be known and used.

The homoeopathic method is very suitable for the treatment

of the 'listed' diseases—sore throat, inflammation of the ear, cystitis, furunculosis, colitis, etc.—but also, and chiefly, for the treatment of a variety of troubles indicative of maladjustment of the organism, malfunction, or poor adaptation. These pathological manifestations are a result of the personality of the patient, the environment in which he is living and the ease or difficulty with which he adapts to it. In all these cases the homoeopathic method is irreplaceable.

Can these manifestations be considered as lying within the domain of medicine? Where is one to draw the line? It is impossible to say. Some people would like to extend the domain of medicine to infinity and medicalise *everything*. Others would like to limit general practice to what is measurable, quantifiable and tangible, and leave the rest to the psychologist or psychoanalyst. I agree, this latter is a reassuring position: you set up little barriers between which you are at home, among people of your own world; you do not set foot outside; in extreme cases, you even deny the existence of the outside world.

'The illness alone is worth studying,' says one side: 'It must be found, tracked down, defined and, if possible, treated.' 'There are no such things as illnesses, there are only sick people', says the other side. And so the dialogue of the deaf starts up again, with one side carrying out further scientific investigations of the most sophisticated kind, and the other remaining lost in artistic flabbiness. Both sets of extremists divorce themselves from reality.

All patients are different—there is no doubt about that—but that does not prevent them occasionally from suffering the same illness. A choleric, explosive, authoritarian person may very well fall downstairs; but so may a timid one. It may or may not be the same staircase—that hardly matters!—but each of them runs the risk of breaking an arm. In that event each of them would need to have an X-ray and to have the arm put in plaster, even though afterwards the difference in their behaviour and character might influence the length of time needed for readjustment, the quality of the healing and the functional recuperation of the broken limb.

For both, the surgeon must perform a completely technical act, and he can well dispense with knowing the characters of his patients. Not so the general practitioner. His knowledge of the way each patient reacts will have a direct effect on the quality of healing and on the amount of medication which will be required—with all the attendant economic or even legal consequences—right from the moment when the injury is experienced by either patient in his own manner.

The case is even clearer if we consider a stomach ulcer. Nowadays everyone recognises the importance of the patient's psychology in the origin of the ulcer. Nevertheless, in the case of a bleeding ulcer radiography, fibroscopy and probably an operation will be necessary. On the other hand, in the case of a patient who complains of cramps at eleven o'clock in the morning and five o'clock in the evening and who says he feels better if he eats something, even if only a little, fibroscopy and radiography will still be necessary to confirm the diagnosis, but the therapy cannot be entirely local. The painful stomach must be seen as just one among a whole range of symptoms, any one of which may, according to the circumstances, be of essential value: poor diet, bad working hours, a submissive or dominant character, difficulty in socialising, and many other things besides. Why should we prefer one of these factors to the others on account of our personal convictions, or what we were once taught or because it is customary to prescribe in accordance with this or that prevailing ideology, or with the volume of publicity from one of the big drug houses?

According to the individual case, the patient's ulcer can be and must be arrested at such and such a stage and treated according to his own reactions; but also, sad to say, according to the capabilities of the doctor and the medical team who are dealing with him.

Numerous children have been brought to me with recurring ailments of the nose and pharynx—colds, bronchitis, inflammation of the ear—which can drag on all the winter. Conventional remedies can be drastic. Yet, even if their illnesses are similar in manifestation, how different these children are and how many solutions could be found if examination was not limited solely to the nasopharyngeal field! Certainly nasopharyngitis is present and it is very real—there is no question of denying that—but why ignore its context? Is it logical and sufficient to look only at the nose and the pharynx? The homoeopathic method taught me that this was not the case; but at the same time it gave me the possibility of working in a holistic manner on the reactivity of the patient, no longer on just a single organ, in the occurrence of nasopharyngitis. Furthermore, I learnt to take note of the fact that certain remote symptoms, apparently having no connection with the sick organ, were far more important in the choice of a homoeopathic remedy than the local symptoms which had been the reason for the consultation.

For example, one day a three-year-old boy was brought to see me. Baby Cadum was a fine specimen with a chubby face, and was very plump—even too plump. According to his parents he was often 'in the dumps'. He ate a lot and slept the whole night through, but perspired freely from the head while doing so, to the extent of dampening his pillow with sweat. He was very quiet, good-natured and easy to look after. Apparently, he was growing well; but regularly, at the slightest cold or whenever it rained—and it does rain a lot in Charente!—he would have bad bouts of fever, reaching 40°C (104°F) within a few hours. He would remain calm in spite of his high temperature, but would perspire more than ever, soaking everything. 'He was just turning into a pool of grease', said his parents.

Every time I was called in, I found an inflamed throat, huge tonsils and large swellings in the neck. Certainly a good dose of antibiotics would quickly put everything right, and the family would be reassured for ten days! I would have liked to take out the tonsils, the real culprits—but I hesitated. Didn't he have some attacks of asthma-like bronchitis a few months ago? And what if he were allergic, like his father with hay-fever or like his grandmother with her asthma? Perhaps what would help on the one hand would do harm on the other? So what was to be done? A course of thermal baths?—but he was much too young. So why not homoeopathy?

The clinical examination was quite normal. The tonsils were

slightly enlarged but became grossly so only during bouts of inflammation; the eardrums were in good condition, and the stethoscope revealed nothing abnormal. In the nose-and-pharynx region, the most significant things were not happening. In accordance with the particular perspective which I had developed, I had to study this child in order to find out his characteristics; his plumpness, the way he behaved like a quiet old man, his copious perspiration, his susceptibility to damp cold, his violent reactions and his rapid recoveries.

To this clinical picture, to all these reactions, there corresponds a homoeopathic remedy called *Calcarea carbonica*. I prescribed this medicine every day for six months. I advised the parents also to keep in reserve a tube of *Belladonna*, and to give him a few pillules every hour after the onset of a feverish attack, adding *Antimonium tartaricum* every half-hour in the case of asthmatic bronchitis. Of course, the child should be brought to see me if everything was not soon right again. During the next few months I was not called in again. The child had had a few little bouts of high temperature which had quickly been brought down by taking *Belladonna*. To the former treatment, I added a few doses of *Thuya*. Three months later, I saw the child again: there was nothing to report. After that, the child had to come back only every six months and have his treatment repeated in September, October and February, for him to continue developing normally, untroubled by winter ills.

Another child was brought to me for the same kind of problems: repeated sore throats, long drawn-out colds, and inflammation of the ear requiring regular draining. He too was three years old, but he was a very different case.

Pale, thin and timid, he crouched on his mother's lap, apprehensive about being at the doctor's again—and, what is more, faced by a new doctor. 'He has always been difficult to bring up,' they told me when I first saw him. 'He has given us a lot of trouble!' As a baby he had been prone to diarrhoea. He had had difficulty in taking milk and his increase in weight, while regular, had been well below normal. Now he was constipated and refused to go to the lavatory. He did not want to eat or ate only when he wanted to, and then only what pleased him. He was timid and nervous, but at the same time domineering and extremely obstinate, a real little family tyrant.

His throat was normal. I found only a few little hard glands in his neck. His chest was narrow, his abdomen distended, his limbs frail. He was chilly, but perspired freely through his feet. When he was ill, the fever came on very slowly; it was not even noticed, and practically never went above 38° or 38.5°C (100.4 or 101.3°F). His nose was always dirty and ran with a thick secretion for days on end. Although, like the former child, this one also showed repeated nasopharyngeal infections, their manifestations were in no way comparable, and neither were the general reactions and behaviour of the two children. For this reason the reactional condition of the second child corresponded to a different homoeopathic remedy: *Silicea*. I advised the mother that, as soon as the 'colds' appeared, she should give him also some pillules of *Ferrum phosphoricum* three or four times a day, supplemented by some pillules of *Pulsatilla* if the nasal secretion appeared.

However, in this particular case, it was evident that the prescription of medicines would probably not be sufficient. It was obvious that a particular kind of relationship had been established between the sickly child and his anxious mother, who was simultaneously over-protective and dismissive. If the circumstances were favourable, if contact was established—not perhaps right at the beginning but after a few consultations—it would be necessary to talk to the mother (or, rather, to let her talk to me) to try to resolve a situation which, according to all the evidence, was not favourable to the child's harmonious development.

'Well then,' you say, 'What is the real value of homoeopathic medicines if a certain amount of psychotherapy has to be used at the same time? Where do you draw the line between the real action of the homoeopathic medicine and the no less genuine therapeutic action achieved by modifying the mother/child relationship? Is the homoeopathic medicine any use at all? Has it any efficacy on its own?'

I think I am qualified to answer 'yes', since I have often

observed its real efficacy when given alone, without the support of any psychotherapy.

For most of the time, as it turned out, it was absolutely impossible to carry out any psychotherapy, because the mother was totally resistant to it or because her defences were too strong, too well organised, for me to be able to modify them in any way at all. In this case, after the simple prescription of medicines, I saw that the child's development began to be modified: his repeated attacks of earache became less frequent, and at the same time his resistance to infection increased. In addition—and this may seem strange to those who have never seen the results of homoeopathic treatment—his character improved, as did his adaptation to the outside world, his behaviour at school and in the family grew less awkward, and the functioning of his digestive system became normal. Nevertheless, in general and if circumstances permit, it is a good thing to intervene in a pathogenic situation which you may have observed in order to try to resolve it.

There is a risk that some people may take these examples as propaganda in favour of homoeopathy. Never mind! It just means that they have not understood or have not wanted to understand anything that I have been saying. Let me repeat yet again, *homoeopathic treatment cannot do everything.*

When a child of the same morphological type, showing the same behaviour, has serious inflammation of the ear, perhaps being even a little deaf, it is necessary at once to open his tympana, put in a grommet and sometimes even take out his adenoids; but why not also prescribe for him *Silicea, Calcarea carbonica* or any other appropriate medicine to avoid possible relapses and, above all, to bring about a progressive modification of the child's general behaviour? Every therapeutic means at our disposal may and must be used whenever the circumstances require it, either alone or in conjunction with another, but certainly without attributing all merits and all virtues to it. Once again we state what seems to us essential: *adapt your action to the situation in force: act on the illness when necessary and on the constitution when necessary; modify the environment, if possible.*

The holistic view presented by the homoeopathic method allows one, among other advantages, always to take these different factors into consideration and to intervene for the best, according to the circumstances.

This conception of illness and patient as a whole is not an abstract, intellectual view, nor an ideological choice; it is a necessity imposed by day-to-day practical medicine, and equally by a knowledge of the action of homoepathic medicines, which, certainly at least in the case of the main medicines, operate on different levels. *Silicea* may act equally well on a localised suppuration (inflammation of the middle ear, a discharging fistula, an encysted abscess) as on a general tendency towards suppuration; but it may also have an effect on the general behaviour, on the psycho-motor development, or on the development of growth and weight. Even if we are unable to *explain* the mechanism, the results are incontestable. *Silicea* may be prescribed just as well for a child with poor development, who is showing behavioural and digestive troubles as described above, with a loving mother who gives him security, as for a child whose troubles have been brought on or made worse by the attitude of an obsessional and over-protective mother. The ideal would be to cause the mother to modify her behaviour; another, and easier, solution would be to help the child not to suffer so much from the consequences.

In my daily practice I meet numerous patients who are allergic to dust, pollen, feathers, or the hair of rabbits or dogs—to name but a few. Here again the problem is to choose the most suitable medicine, even if the nature of the illness differs from case to case. If these patients have a particular, very definite allergy, the best thing to do is to avoid the allergen; but how are you to prevent a farmer who is allergic to chaff from going into his barn or stable? Certainly you can help him by diminishing his sensitivity—that is to say, accustoming him to stand increasing doses of chaff. But this solution, 'specific desensitisation', is not necessarily the best, since the patient is rarely allergic to chaff alone. Most often, as this allergy improves, one sees a second one developing proportionately, and so it all starts again for two or three years with an injection every week or fortnight.

It might also be tempting to work on the constitutional background of this poor farmer suffering the injustices of such an infirmity: his neighbours, after all, are perfectly able to go into *their* barns without sneezing! The allergist and immunologist could obviously give a partial answer to this question, which, behind its apparent simplicity, touches on an extremely complex problem.

Yet, after all, apart from changing his job and desensitisation, there is not much to suggest, since the doctor does not know and cannot work on the particular constitutional background. According to orthodox medical opinion, nothing can be done until this background *per se* has been discovered and defined. 'And yet,' says the homoeopath, 'aspirin was certainly used before we knew how it worked.' Indeed, at the beginning it was prescribed as a result of a completely ludicrous idea, derived from the doctrine of signatures as advanced by Paracelsus. Facts are more important than theories, and the latter very often have but a fleeting existence. This background, which is not yet recognised biologically, may possibly be known in its clinical reality.

The farmer in question—an active, jolly fellow and a big eater—had had all sorts of spots ever since he was born: eczema as a child, boils at twenty, and now 'itchy' patches and fungus between his toes. The bouts of sneezing and the unending colds had begun appearing three or four years ago.

Among these symptoms, which were so ordinary as to appear negligible, a homoeopathic doctor could find enough material to recognise a certain type of reaction indicating a particular constitutional background on which it is possible to work by prescribing *Nux vomica* and *Sulphur*. Quite often the homoeopathic doctor finds that the intervals between the crises increase while the crises themselves diminish in intensity. It is important to stress that *Nux vomica* and *Sulphur* are not allergy medicines, but medicines for certain patients who have, among other things, an allergy which manifests in a particular way.

The farmer's cousin also came to see me—he too was

allergic. He had been astonished by the results his cousin had achieved, and wondered if the same medicines would do the same for him; but he was very thin and quiet, a chilly person. I did not even have to ask him about that. It was June, yet he was wearing a thick hand-knitted pullover of good country wool and corduroy trousers, and had his cap on his knees—indeed, it was obvious that he would rather have kept it on his head except out of respect for me.

He could not remember ever having not been ill. As a baby he had had eczema; as a child bronchitis and asthma. He even had to be sent for a cure. He did get better after a few years and he finally lost his asthma; but he remained delicate. 'You cannot imagine what it is like.' He would get tired by nothing at all; he was always like that. He was never hungry, so how could he have any resistance? 'Just between you and me doctor, do you really think things will ever get any better?'

The said 'things' were the eczema on his legs, his fits of sneezing which had begun two or three years before, and then the asthma, which had come back and which started up every night at about one o'clock in the morning. 'I even have to get up to open the window! You see I am stifled when it is shut and yet I simply can't stand the cold; so I have a big blanket and wrap myself up in it. This performance goes on every night. It's no joke for me ... nor for the wife either. Do you think you can do anything for me? After all this time, I hardly believe anyone could help, but it might be worth a try ... '

All that would be enough to send a technical doctor to sleep; just a string of symptoms without any apparent significance at all. On the other hand, what was important to note was his immunoglobulin. However, it was much less simple to determine the treatment and put it into practice. Should one opt for desensitisation? With which allergen should one begin? Should the patient avoid contact with the allergens—by living in a hermetically sealed box?

There remained corticotherapy, with all its advantages and disadvantages. Only an unscrupulous or incompetent doctor would lightly embark, without having thought deeply, on this therapy, which should be kept as a last resort to be used only in extreme cases where all other means have failed. Before deciding on this solution, might it not be better to consider another, simpler one, which in addition would be without risk?

Any doctor with a knowledge of the homoeopathic *materia medica* knows the toxic effect of arsenic and the therapeutic effect of a dilution of *Arsenicum album*. He knows, too, the effect of other medicines—*Psorinum*, for example, which could equally well be used in a similar situation.

I did indeed use them in this case—and in many others, too—and the results I obtained encouraged me to continue on these lines. All the same, it should not be thought that I have cured all of my patients!

So, for twenty years I have been using homoeopathic medicines. I observe and study my patients according to the homoeopathic method. When I prescribe for them I base my choice on the law of analogy, and I get very good results; but I confess that I do not really understand what is happening. I do not know how my medicines work, and for this reason I get into great difficulties when I argue with my colleagues, who are not homoeopaths and who would like to find some logical explanation as to how my therapy works.

Even if they see the good results and they show confidence in me by regularly sending me patients, I am convinced that most of them think that homoeopathic medicine is ineffective, that it is nothing but a common placebo. The cure is achieved only because I have the time to listen to my patients; because my medicines, with their Latin names, have a certain mystery which attracts and intrigues the patients; and perhaps, too, because I am outside conventional medicine and my fees are higher than theirs!

It would be easy to object that the mechanisms by which the majority of orthodox medicines work are not known either, and that the results of their use vary according to different individuals and their constitutional backgrounds. However, the orthodox medicines are much more numerous than the homoeopathic ones, and their interactions are so obvious that large works are devoted to the matter of incompatibilities, a phenomenon unknown in homoeopathy.

Some chance meetings—and my great friendship with the director of one of the drug houses—have given me the opportunity, during the last eight years, to cut down on my medical work and to undertake, in parallel, a certain number of experiments on animals. I am trying, like many who have preceded me in this line, to show the real and measurable action of homoeopathic medicines. This action is indeed real and measurable, and can be reproduced in precise experimental conditions, yet it is constantly called into question, the most vehement critics being those who know least about the subject.

If the action of homoeopathic medicines is unfortunately still too often contested, it is more for reasons of prerogative and defence of territory than for scientific concern. In fact, the resistance is at this height in medical circles and much less among scientists. A scientist, indeed, never feels that his personality is being attacked when he is confronted with a new fact, even if this fact clashes with his ideas and startles him. He tries to verify it or he does all he can to refute it, but he never rejects it outright. The attitude towards homoeopathy among biologists, physicists and pharmacologists, to name but a few, is friendly, and collaboration always proves possible, even if discussion is sometimes heated and no quarter is given!

At the present time numerous research programmes are under way. They are being carried out by homoeopaths as well as by orthodox scientists, thanks to close cooperation between the various researchers who in university laboratories define the scope of researches, draw up the protocols and carry them out.

This is not the case in those medical circles where the arguments advanced against homoeopathy are purely emotional in nature. Every discussion, which one had hoped would be serious, degenerates rapidly. Each person, whether a partisan of orthodox therapy or not, tries to defend a certain number of preconceptions and immediately turns the debate into an oratorical jousting-match, in which he considers only his personal position, forgetting that the *facts* are there and that it is those facts alone which should be discussed.

Homoeopathy

I really do not know why it is that homoeopathy seems able to find only ardent and uncompromising defenders, who accept everything without criticism, or adversaries who persist in being blind and deaf to every argument which is put forward. At any rate, I would gratify me considerably if this book could be the point of departure for a truly objective and critical discussion about what homoeopathy is and what it could be if it emerged from the realm of polemics in which it is too often confined.

CHAPTER III

Homoeopathy

INTRODUCTION TO HOMOEOPATHY

If you read the currently available works on general medical topics you will find that most authors, whether or not they are in favour of homoeopathy, have made snap judgements and have lacked proper information about the subject. To avoid subsequent confusion or risk of mistaken interpretation we should at the outset give a clear definition of homoeopathy. A dictionary definition that we are happy to endorse reads: 'Homoeopathy is a method of treating the sick by the use of minute doses of a drug which, in a healthy person, would produce symptoms similar to those of the illness being treated.'

This method of treatment is founded on two criteria which define its area of application and the limits thereto: use of the *law of similars* (sometimes called the *law of analogy*) when choosing the remedy, and the prescription of the remedy in minute reactive doses, *infinitesimal doses*.

Homoeopathy was born at the end of the 18th century. At the outset it was purely a therapeutic technique, subsequently becoming a theory of medicine also, based on empirically observed facts in a series of experiments as rigorous as they are generally ill known. From ancient times doctors had observed that in some cases there is a resemblance between the toxic and therapeutic effects of certain substances. The writings of Hippocrates make mention of two complementary therapeutic

67

methods: the therapy of opposites and the therapy of similars. While the former engendered considerable support and so came to dominate the medical world, the latter was generally forgotten, being used only by certain alchemical doctors who dealt in analogies that were often more formal than real.

Only at the end of the 18th century were its possibilities again subjected to study and brought together as a coherent system of treatment. It came about somewhat by chance. Translating a book from English, Christian Hahnemann (1755-1843) became aware of a fact that seemed strange to him. In the book, mention was made of the fact that quinquina poisoning could trigger an outbreak of a feverish condition identical in all respects to malaria, which disease was usually cured by taking a decoction of quinquina bark. In modern terms, of course, we realise that the active agent in both the poisoning and the decoction is quinine.

He then took an experimentally rigorous step. Following to the letter the advice of the great Swiss physiologist Albrecht von Haller, that the action of each medicament should be studied on a healthy man before being prescribed for a patient, Hahnemann decided to see whether the statement in the English medical work was tur. He took a fixed dose of quinquina and observed the appearance of feverish symptoms which resembled in every degree those which quinine normally cures.

Luckily for the future development of homoeopathy, Hahnemann had a particular sensitivity to quinine. Although today its effects and certain of its mechanisms are well known, this sensitivity is relatively rare. Hahnemann's experiment was roundly criticised by several authors who, having repeated it and not obtained similar results, abandoned their investigations and thoroughly condemned a method which went so against normal practice. However, Hahnemann was not alone in observing the phenomenon. Bretonneau de Tours indicated this several years later in a medical and surgical journal of the time. He published case-histories of a number of patients who showed therapeutic intolerance to quinine. Some of these observations appeared in Trousseau and Pidoux's *Traité de matière médicale* of 1858.

The happy success of his experiment, combined with his relentless curiosity, led Hahnemann to research further into the medical literature. He discovered that numerous observations of the same type had already been made in relation to other substances, and these he collected all together in a bibliographical catalogue which he then published.

From the diverse observations he established a working hypothesis and an experimental method. The hypothesis is simple: 'Medicaments cure the sick only by virtue of their ability to make people sick, and they cure only those illnesses whose symptoms are similar to those they themselves can produce in a healthy organism.'

The initial method of experiment was based solely on observation of acute or chronic toxicology; but Hahnemann quickly defined and described an extremely precise method of study so that he might obtain what he called 'a medicinal pathogenesis'. By this he meant the sum of symptoms created by the repeated taking of a given substance either in toxic or subtoxic dose over a variable length of time. In the course of these experiments he produced detailed accounts of the action of the principal medicinal substances which were used empirically at that time. These accounts formed the basis of the *Homoeopathic Materia Medica*, a compilation of the potential therapeutic action of medicinal substances used by homoeopathic doctors.

When he considered that his knowledge was wide enough and sufficiently supported, he undertook a careful series of practical therapeutic trials, prescribing for the patients entrusted to him weak doses of medicaments with whose toxic effects in strong doses he was well acquainted. He observed that a number of cures took place.

After ten years of experiment and observation he arrived at a definition of a law of treatment which for the first time in medical history introduced a certain amount of logic and strictness in prescription things previously lacking in the empirical and confused medicine of the time. This law, known as the law of similars—'*Similia similibus curentur*' or 'like cures like' is the basic rule of homoeopathic treatment and the sole criterion is defining this method's field of action. It found contemporary confirmation in the work of Jenner and subsequently in certain of Pasteur's observations.

The law did not spring ready-formed from the mind of an enlightened being, as some would have it. Far from it: it is the conclusion drawn from a series of careful and precise experiments. The fortuitous observation of a fact; the search for other similar facts; and the establishment of a hypothesis and an experimental method to verify the hypothesis.

Homoeopathy claims neither to be a dogma nor the one and only valid method of treatment, but simply to be a single therapeutic possibility which is valuable in certain cases. This was what Hahnemann himself thought. He was against all attempts to be categorical about things and expressed his law in subtle terms, deliberately using the subjunctive *curentur* in preference to the present indicative *curantur*.

From the outset he had conceived of homoeopathy as a technique of therapy, but very soon, relying both on practice and on clinical and experimental observations, he constructed a medical doctrine in which one can recognise, mixed in with his original ideas, the influence of certain concepts then current —particularly the vitalist theories which would find their full expression with Basthez and Montpellier.

It is clear that this theoretical conception, in the precise terms in which it was spelled out, cannot today be accepted uncritically. It is not and never has been, except to a few people, a sacred dogma. It is merely an attempted explanation; one working hypothesis among several of great interest, but always subject to change, as knowledge develops.

The theory, established in an epoch of medical history very different from our own, fits perfectly into the sum of contemporary medical thinking. The central essence concerns taking the individual, judged as a unique being, fully into consideration. The hypothesis also conceives of illness as a momentary modification of normal physiological functioning under the influence of a variety of causes, of both internal and external origin. This is the crystallisation of homoeopathy.

In summary, then, as a therapy, homoeopathy is founded on

the two criteria we have met: the law of similars (for the choice of medicament) and the habitual prescription of infinitesimal doses prepared using especially laid-down techniques. We feel that *any* therapeutic technique can and should be of interest to a doctor, particularly if it helps him in his daily practice.

Homoeopathy is also a medical concept: it is neither exclusive nor definitive, and it is not, as some people seem to think, opposed to current medical theory—quite the opposite. It has the advantage of being situated at the intersection of medical science and the humanities, bringing an original perspective to the problems of health and sickness. It is a personalised form of medicine which brings its interest to bear on an overall understanding of the sick individual in his environment, and of the personal character of his morbid reactions.

This well balanced concept may allow a widening of the field of therapy and be of real use at a period when greater and greater specialisation and the accelerating development of an often inhuman technicality risk the essential rôle of the doctor being forgotten. This is particularly true in the case of the general practitioner, the poor relation of medical practice.

AN ORIGINAL METHOD OF THERAPY

Homoeopathy as a therapy is founded on a simple method which has been fully codified since the end of the 18th century; the therapeutic technique is still applicable, without modification, today. It remains a perfectly usable working tool both in the realm of practical medicine and in the realm of basic research. Designed from the outset to give structure to an entirely empirical therapy, the homoeopathic method was the first logical attempt at analytical pharmacology and therapy. Consideration of this method, worked out in detail so as to apply as simply as possible the law of similars when choosing a medicine, enables us to give a satisfactory definition of the scope of homoeopathy, its characteristics, its potential and its limitations.

Homoeopathy

It is a system of treatment which works by analogy and can only be put into practice by comparing two clinical pictures: that of the patient and that which comes from experimenting with medicinal substances on a healthy person. Hahnemann's careful codifying of this method of therapy from the outset means that the therapy is still perfectly valid today; his only aim in establishing it was to put the law of similars into practice.

To prescribe in accordance with the law of analogy one should, for any given illness, know on the one hand the apparent manifestations and on the other the action of the medicinal substances. One should then compare the clinical picture, as observed in the patient, with the experimental clinical picture as it unfolds in the experimenter's body.

This method has three clearly defined aspects: *an experimental aspect*, which produces evidence of the action of the medicinal substances in the experimenter; *an observational aspect*, in which the patient's symptoms are codified; and *a therapeutic aspect*, giving the rules for prescribing medicines in each clinical case.

These three aspects are of interest to pharmacists and pharmacologists, to practising doctors and to basic scientific researchers. The observational and therapeutic aspects will be studied in the chapter dealing with medical consultation; for the moment we will concentrate on the experimental aspect, which is the real basis of the homoeopathic method.

An Original Experiment
The originality of homoeopathy lies in the idea of experimenting with medicinal substances in the healthy person. How was this done?

Starting from the hypothesis that a substance whose effects on a healthy person were clearly known could be used as a medicine, Hahnemann perfected a technique designed to study this activity.

His first concern was to define precisely the origin and method of preparation of the experimental substance. Then, according to strictly defined guidelines, he observed the effects on a number of volunteers. To do this the substance was given in varying subtoxic doses to each of the experimenters, who then had to note carefully the manner of appearance and development of any symptoms. The mass of results obtained, taken together, contributed to the building-up of the *Homoeopathic Materia Medica*, an essential reference work for any doctor practising homoeopathy.

Unlike classical *materia medica*, which limit their study to the physicochemical properties and natural history of medicinal substances, the *Homoeopathic Materia Medica* additionally describes the action of the substances on a healthy person. Therein lies its originality.

For each medicament three kinds of symptoms are listed: toxic symptoms, 'pathogenic' symptoms and 'clinical' symptoms. Acute or chronic toxic symptoms, triggered by accidental poisoning, are well known to toxicologists. Pathogenic symptoms are observed in experiments carried out according to the Hahnemann techniques. They are of the greatest interest, and are the most characteristic of the homoeopathic method, as they are not studied in classical research. Clinical symptoms, though not pathogenic, may be treated by empirical use of the medicinal substance.

These experiments on the action of the various medicaments on people, coupled with an original interpretation of their results, led to two fundamental ideas from which we can learn a lot, but which are currently paid too little attention.

An enemy can become a friend

Each substance triggers particular symptoms in each individual being tested. When a substance is given in sufficient doses, it produces in everyone symptoms which are characteristic of that substance. These manifestations are specific to the action of the medicament and are localised in certain tissues, organs or functions of the body. They are immensely useful to the doctor in the choice of his prescription.

The basic principle of homoeopathic treatment is extremely simple: a substance which in toxic or subtoxic dose produces a

73

pattern of clinical, biological or anatomo-pathological symptoms may, after experiment and in an infinitesimal dilution, become the medicine with which a condition with similar symptoms may be treated.

Arsenic, for example, tends to trigger skin troubles, with the appearance of hyperkeratosis; phosphorus causes damage to liver cells; *Nux vomica* contains strychnine, which acts as a poison to the nervous system. Yet in minute doses all three can be used therapeutically. Knowledge of this polarity of action is vitally important to homoeopaths. By the law of similars, infinitesimal doses of arsenic can be used to treat dry eczema; of phosphorus to treat viral or alcohol-induced hepatitis; and of *Nux vomica* to treat nervous complaints, particularly hyperexcitability and spasm.

This resemblance of symptoms probably masks a similarity between the mechanisms involved. The law of similars, having shown itself to be of prime importance as far as treatment is concerned, could play an equally useful rôle in basic research. However, one should remember that the law of similars is not always verifiable. Nonetheless, it provides an extremely interesting method of 'prospecting', of experimenting systematically on laboratory animals.

Though it is often difficult to extrapolate from animals to man, some fundamental processes—phenomena associated with inflammation, for instance—are virtually identical.

Each reacts acording to his ability

The second idea, equally if not more important, is as follows: some people are more susceptible than others to certain substances. The concept of individual sensitivity or individual reaction follows from the pathogenic experiments carried out by the homoeopaths.

If, in an experiment, the substance under investigation is given in a relatively strong dose, all test cases show identical symptoms. If, on the other hand, the substance is given in frequently repeated, very small doses, it produces visible signs only in certain subjects. These particularly receptive people are called 'sensitive individuals'.

This fact, well known to homoeopaths, seemed strange to toxicologists, who had in general had only the opportunity of observing the effects of acute or chronic poisoning after the intake of relatively high doses of the toxic substance. Today the phenomenon is better understood by the medical world, which is constrained more and more to study the harmful effects of the various pollutants in our environment: it has been noticed how only certain individuals show lack of tolerance to the various kinds of pollution.

In these observations can be found the origin of homoeopathic typology and characterology.

Minute examination of these hypersensitive individuals has allowed the description of a number of morphological or characterological symptoms, and thanks to this it is possible to identify subjects reacting exceptionally to one substance or another.

For example, a lank, pale easily tired person will react more readily to the prescription of phosphorus or its salts, while a squat, solid-set round-faced person with large square hands will react more favourably to calcium or its salts. An aggressive, hyperactive man will be more susceptible to the action of *Nux vomica*, while a distrustful, reflective introverted type will react only to *Lycopodium*. Another type again—meticulous, anxious and shivery—will be susceptible only to arsenic.

Homoeopathic characterology and typology, the fruit of long observation, are described in the same terms as classical typology and characterology: thus one can recognise the patient sensitive to *Nux vomica* as the Emotive-Active-Primary and the patient sensitive to *Lycopodium* as the Emotional-Non-active-Secondary. As well as producing these evaluations and establishing constants, as is done in classical medicine, they bring an important additional factor: a therapeutic action to be taken immediately the symptoms of imbalance appear.

Established on a solid experimental basis, the homoeopathic method provides the doctor with a large range of medicaments which he can study and use in many instances, ranging from functional maladjustments to a lesion.

While it has, until recently, been limited only to the clinical study of immediately observable symptoms it can, at the level of fundamental research, be used in a systematic way to examine the biological, anatomopathological or metabolic manifestations of acute or chronic poisoning; and then to compare them with the biological, anatomopathological or metabolic manifestations typical of certain illnesses for which no treatment may yet have been suggested. This work will be in the same general line as that of pharmacologists, whose basic objectives are on the one hand to determine the area and method of action of each substance and, on the other, to study the individual sensitivity of each patient to a medicinal substance in terms of his genetic constitution and his enzymatic stock. Is the hope that one day a fruitful research project will be carried out jointly, thanks to a more open attitude of mind, too idealistic? We think not, believing that this hope of ours must be shared by others.

A DIFFERENT CONCEPT OF MEDICINE

From the very beginning, homoeopathic medicine has shown itself to be a method of observation and experiment founded on an original theoretical basis. Using empirical observation followed by experiment, Hahnemann, from the end of the 18th century (a time when medicine was in great confusion) defined a precise system of treatment and drew up a theory of medicine based on two essential ideas: the individual as a whole, and dynamism. These two concepts fit very well indeed into the body of theories accepted by the medical establishment.

The individual as a whole

In the first edition of *The Organon*, Hahnemann clearly indicated the need to study the totality of symptoms shown by the patient for 'only the totality of symptoms can reveal the image of the illness'. Ahead of his time, he advised a purely phenomenological study of the illness so far as it is accessible to the senses; from this viewpoint he insisted on collating all the apparent symptoms in an attempt better to understand the body's upset.

For Hahnemann, the organism is a whole and no one part may arbitrarily be isolated or granted undue importance during observation. But equally, as far as he was concerned, the organism has to be treated as an integral part of its environment. He advises that, when examining the patient, proper attention should be paid to the conditions in which he lives and his relations with those with whom he lives.

If any function is isolated from the whole there is the risk of error, on account of the large number of interrelationships of all sorts between the various parts of an individual person ...

The various parts of the body are interdependent and form an indivisible whole, as far as both the body's sensations and its functions are concerned. One cannot imagine a mouth ulcer or simple whitlow without a background deficiency; that is to say, without the patient's general condition having played a part ...

One cannot really imagine a genuine therapy which does not take the general state of the body into consideration ...

In each individual case of illness, the sum of the symptoms should be the doctor's chief concern and the sole object of his attentions, and his aim should be to eliminate the totality by his intervention, thereby producing a cure and transforming the patients state from illness into health ...

One cannot be clearer than that.

In Hahnemann's writings the idea of totality or wholeness has two sources, one philosophical and the other experimental. His way of thinking is in the hippocratic tradition and in the general line of the formulated concepts of medicine.

Had not Hippocrates indicated that the individual should be seen as the sum of his reactions, which themselves depended greatly on his temperament and on the environment in which he lived? For this reason Hahnemann advised proper study of the background, both physical and psychological, of the patient, as well as of the general conditions of his life.

77

This philosophical position was then, as Hahnemann formulated his *Homoeopathic Materia Medica*, confirmed by observation—observation of the patient, of course, but more importantly of the action of medicinal substances on human beings. Such experiments showed him that, if the symptoms were noted with care and without preconceptions, the progressive action of the experimental substance was seen in all the body's functions, even if it seemed to be more clearcut in the case of one organ than in that of another.

A reading of the *Homoeopathic Materia Medica* demonstrates effectively that, if certain remedies appear to show a polarity of action on certain organs, in reality it is the individual as a whole who is modified. In order to bring this about, though, it is necessary to listen to everything, to examine everything, instead of arbitrarily focussing attention on particular symptoms.

A particular example reveals the richness and value of this method of total observation.

Mercury poisoning is well known and is described in all the works on toxicology. However, only the physical symptoms are summarised. Hahnemann and his pupils described, as an advance warning of mercury poisoning, in addition to the localised symptoms a complete pattern of psychological signs, the most important of which were irritability and the tendency to become angry. Occupational health doctors in Britain have recently carried out an investigation into the early warning symptoms of mercury poisoning, in order to be able to detect as rapidly as possible those workers who are affected. Enquiries amongst the wives of those patients recognised through normal biological examinations as suffering from poisoning revealed a strange but manifest fact: in the two or three months preceding biological symptoms of poisoning, they had observed a character change in their husbands, and an unaccustomed tendency to flare up angrily.

This symptom, known to all homoeopaths, could just as well have been known to toxicologists had they bothered to research subjective symptoms as well as measurable objective ones.

It is a characteristic of our time that only what is

measurable is regarded as scientific, leaving everything else languishing in the shadows. One has to recognise the value of the scientific method, which has led to important discoveries, but carried to absurd lengths it becomes dangerous, for this way of determining what is and what is not real sets arbitrary limits to the scope of investigation.

Today, the two key concepts—of the unity and of the individuality of a person—mean that the patient cannot be divorced from the illness. An objective and subjective, somatic and psychological, study of all the symptoms can hardly be criticised. Indeed, after a long period in which it has been concerned solely with the anatomical malady, and while still maintaining this approach, orthodox medicine is nevertheless increasingly turning its attention to psychological phenomena and to an overall appreciation of the patient. Specialisation, carried to extremes—which has led to treating the individual as a collection of little bits, and to studying each of his systems apart from the others—has finally engendered a healthy reaction, which has drawn attention to the unity of each human being. J. Delay has remarked:

> The psychosomatic movement seeks to replace a medicine of organs, which has become more and more specialised and localised, with a general medicine of the organism. It gives prime importance to the role of the constitution, so renewing links with the hippocratic tradition, which considers illness, less as an accident or an inevitable process which is to some extent unrelated to the patient, more as intimately related to his reactions and ultimately to his nature.

In a recent book H. P. Klotz says that, for him, 'the real general practitioner is someone who knows how to place a particular symptom or condition in the general context of his patient's life and health. He is a man who, in all cases, makes a general synthesis and sees the patient as a whole.' The patient at each consultation represents not only an immediate and localised problem but also a totality and a history. The doctor's rôle is to put the malfunction of one organ into the context of the whole body, to relate it to the general development of the patient's personality, and to reintegrate all this into the patient's social background. The general practitioner has to 'substitute for the simplistic and mechanistic theory of single causality the complex dialectic of multi factored causality'.

We could give many quotations on this subect, for the concept of the totality of the individual is very much to the fore. Further quotations could equally embrace medical practice or fundamental bilogical research. They would not, however, add anything to our purpose, which is simply to make it understood that homoeopathy is no anachronism but, on the contrary, extremely modern.

Dynamism

The other idea basic to homoepathic therapy lays itself even wider open to criticism, especially if improperly understood or confined to the narrow framework in which it was originally expressed. In Hahnemann's terms dynamism was a form of vitalism: it was an explanation of the transition from a state of illness to a state of health through modification of the vital force.

This idea is, at best, a tentative explanation of some merit in the 18th century. As F. Jacob says in his book *Logic of Living* (*La logique du vivant*), 'vitalism comes into play only after observation; it is an aid not to seeing but to interpretation'. This is exactly the intellectual step forward taken by Hahnemann. After carrying out objective experiments, he tried to explain the re-establishment of health by the action of a 'medicinal energy' on 'morbid energy'.

To do justice to these ideas of energy, which are at the heart of homoeopathic theory, we should put them in their context.

At the time, they provided the only possible explanation of the functional modes characteristic of life as well as a way to react against the abuses of cartesian mechanics. To cite Jacob again, 'Recourse to a vital principle is a product of one of the foundations of biology, the necessity to separate living creatures from inanimate objects, and to base this distinction not on matter, whose unity is known, but on forces. Vitalism is thus as essential to the birth of biology as mechanicalism was to the classical age.' Nowadays, we can understand mechanistics in a different way, for two new concepts have been added: 'Today, living beings appear as the focus of a triple flow of matter, energy and information. At its simplest biology is able to recognise a flow of matter, but, in place of the other two, one has to have recourse to a special force.'

P. Cornillot wrote recently (*Autrement*, September 1977)

Since all living organisms are necessarily in a state of permanent change, the idea of health cannot be understood biologically except in terms of a dynamic equilibrium maintained within the limits of natural compensation. Illness represents, then, an imbalance in the system which exceeds the possibilities of compensation, and introduces a new state whose development can be limited and which can be reduced naturally through the defence mechanism or which can be led to an irreversible deterioration of the biological mechanisms, until death ensues.

This approach lets us understand that therapy can act in tandem with the natural biological mechanisms of compensation, either in seeking to destroy or reduce the pathogenic effects of a causal agent, or in seeking to make good the vital biological functions which have temporarily or permanently been altered.

This concept parallels the homoeopathic approach to health and sickness. For a homoeopath, illness is simply a modification of the individual norm which one has first to study and come to know—and health is the maintenance of a dynamic equilibrium within limits which vary from person to person. Thanks to external or internal influences, this equilibrium may be modified, at first imperceptibly, until various indications—symptoms that indicate disorganisation—demonstrate clearly that disorganisation has become real, measurable and quantifiable; now that it has become significant, it is accorded due consideration.

It is for this reason that the homeopathic doctor attaches such importance to knowledge, through long, precise and detailed questioning, of the general behaviour pattern of his patients and the most likely fashion in which they will act or react.

In certain illnesses, as the result of a massive and brutal attack, serious physical manifestations occur and evolve in a stereotyped manner, requiring equally stereotyped treatment. Cerebrospinal meningitis and acute tuberculosis are two examples. Treatment has to be codified and uniform, whoever the individual patient. It goes without saying that these illnesses are outside the domain of homoeopathy. But other illnesses—the majority, in fact—are difficult to classify. They set in motion regulatory mechanisms which are common to all people (and often to animals as well), and this allows the opportunity for reproducible scientific study within certain experimental limits. But then these general regulatory mechanisms are modified from one person to another because of individual modes of response. These depend both on the genetic constitution of each individual and on the functional relationship which the genotype has established with the environment through fortuitous events which, during the course of an individual's liife, have or have not allowed the expression of his or her genetic potential.

These 'functional illnesses, so-called because they are not measurable or quantifiable, comprise the true and important realm of homoeopathy. In addition, they are popular targets of contemporary research. But this, when carried out in the classical manner, remains purely conceptual and leads only to theoretical solutions. For this reason it is, unfortunately, not adapted to the improvement of therapy: the practising doctor remains stuck between two extreme solutions, that of psychotherapy or that of brutal and often, because of its secondary effects, harmful treatment.

Between these two extremes, however, there is an immense area in which reactive therapy, able to modify, regulate and balance the sick, so allowing them to live to the best that their individual norm allows, may act. This therapy is homoeopathy.

A PARTICULAR TYPE OF CONSULTATION

Every doctor has a certain number of problems with consultations: hearing the patient's complaint, understanding his requirements, instituting a dialogue, carefully noting the symptoms described and the symptoms observed, making a synthesis of these disparate elements, establishing a diagnosis, instituting a treatment, and then explaining this treatment to the patient so that he will be aware that his message has been received and understood, that diagnosis has taken place, and that the most appropriate therapy has been started.

Listening to and Examining the Patient

From the outset, the patient produces a varied symptomatology, most often centred on one symptom which is particularly bothering him. This symptomatology is usually rich and apparently complicated, for it is expressed in direct, personal terms which bear little relation to medical jargon. The doctor listens, observes behaviour, attitude and bodily signals, and then starts to sort out the symptoms according to the interest each holds for him.

Listening is the most important part of the medical act. It allows the establishment of the initial picture, the picture of the illness as felt and lived by the patient; from listening the doctor gains his first impression of the relative importance of the disorder's lesional, functional and psychosomatic aspects. The picture is likely to be rich in subjective, often graphic or unusual, described symptoms which might seem not to have any value. They are, however, vital to a subsequent understanding of the patient, and are of undeniable value in the choice of medicament or medicaments prescribed.

First one studies the illness which brought the patient to the consultation, bearing in mind that it is only one element, and not necessarily the most important. One notes the patient's medical history in detail, seeking in articular for the initial symptoms and the conditions under which they appeared, how they developed, and then the current symptoms, detailing for each the particular conditions which make it better or worse. Next one enquires about the patient's previous history and heredity—that is to say, any illnesses which he, his father, his mother, his brother or his sisters may have had. Finally, one questions him about all the other symptoms he displays, in whatever sphere, giving particular attention to his principal characteristics, his way of reacting to outside events, and the way in which he fits into his social and family milieux.

One then moves on to an objective examination, looking for all the classical signs (palpation, percussion, etc.), and arranging any relevant secondary examination (X-rays, laboratory examination of specimens) which shows itself to be necessary. It would be useless to detail further this technical phase, which should be gone through by every doctor, whether homoeopathic or not. It goes without saying that only through this technical examination will the existence of a physical injury be disclosed or disproved.

The clinical examination is completed by a more specific examination: the search for objective signs according to homoeopathic semiology (morphological symptoms, for instance) so as best to determine the 'sensitive type' to which the patient belongs.

The Symptoms as a Whole

In this way a summary of all the symptoms presented by the patient, subjective and objective, psychological and somatic, is established. A homoeopathic consultation is, in fact, a psychosomatic consultation in the true sense of the term, for it is concerned simultaneously with psychological and somatic symptoms, giving undue weight to neither. The balance of importance depends on the patient and his circumstances. It would be stupid, during either observation or interpretation, to dogmatically give preference to one over the other.

There are cases of angina pectoris which accompany psychological problems (often triggered by violent emotion), just as there are psychological problems associated with a classic example of arteriosclerosis. Some vesicular cases have bursts of critical hepatic colic enhanced or aggravated by the way in which they live; in other patients these crises are associated with chronic cholecystitis due to the formation of gall stones. The localised symptoms of hepatic colic will be exactly the same; the accompanying symptoms will be totally different, and the decision in favour of medical or surgical intervention will depend more on an analysis of the patient as a whole than on a purely local study of the vesicular condition.

Since the illness and the patient together comprise a unity, it seems to us entirely illogical to separate, arbitrarily, the illness from its context. Nor does it seem logical to isolate artificially the significant symptoms of a known illness while, on the other hand, ignoring the significant symptoms of the patient's general reaction.

This taking in hand of the whole individual, this open, non-exclusive study of the entire range of symptoms, this concept of the individual as a whole and the holistic view of the human being as inseparable from his or her environment (far more often talked about than actually put into practice) is frequently rejected—amid many misunderstandings, arguments between different schools of thought, and, more important, harmful or useless therapeutic treatment.

In the case of a feverish patient, why limit your observation to taking his temperature (a measurable symptom)? Why not also observe if the patient is pale and sweating or if, on the other hand, he is congested, excitable, anxious and suffering from dry skin? The fever is common to both types of patient, but their mode of reaction is different.

These secondary symptoms have no place in classical treatment which, in the absence of a recognised aetiology and deprived of the means of diagnosis, limits itself to prescribing a febrifuge. Yet, for the homoeopathic physician, who is more interested in the reactions than in the symptoms in isolation, they are extremely valuable, for they will guide his choice of medication. For the first case he would prescribe a dilution of *Belladonna;* for the second a dilution of *Aconite.*

No apparent logical connection between symptoms of (a) high temperature, sweating and prostration and (b) high temperature, agitation and anxiety can be established. Yet these reactive syndromes exist: one encounters them in clinical practice. Nevertheless, they have yet to be recognised or studied by pharmacologists.

Belladonna or aconite poisoning causes the relevant symptoms. So why do small doses of these substances effect a cure? At present we do not know, but our temporary ignorance is not sufficient reason by itself to justify the attitudes of indifference or rejection which the prospect of treating fevers in this way arouses. On the contrary, it would seem more scientific to us, once one has objectively noted the facts, to look for an explanation (or explanations) of these phenomena in terms of the body's initial defence mechanisms.

Homoeopathic doctors have noticed that certain groups of symptoms are characteristic of the toxic or subtoxic action of a variety of substances. It has been established, in a systematic and reproducible way, that the prescription of minute doses of these substances can give genuine therapeutic benefit. This is more than enough to justify homoeopathic medical practice. But the fact that such phenomena can be shown to occur does not make it any less desirable to study and reveal the mechanism underlying them. Such investigation lies in the realm of pharmacology, and it is up to the pharmacologists to carry out systematic research in this hitherto apparently neglected field.

The Grouping Symptoms
Such a collection of symptoms is not sufficient to establish a diagnosis and decide on a treatment. Diagnosis depends on choosing the most significant symptoms and grouping them into a coherent whole. The collected symptoms are not all of equal importance; in each clinical case they have, therefore, to be classified and coordinated.

Every manifestation of sickness is dependent upon both the background (that is to say, an external agent) and the constitution (that is to say, individual predispositions), *and* on their reciprocal relationship. Certain symptoms are born of a well defined illness, others of a clear aetiology, yet others of the patient's individual reaction. The value all is not absolute, but relative in terms of the whole. Only by examining all the factors, free of theoretical conditions, can one hope to establish the relative value of each.

In some cases, rare in daily practice, the overall symptoms correspond to an illness perfectly defined by its aetiology, its particular manifestations and its development. Whether such an illness should be treated classically or homoeopathically depends upon the circumstances.

More often than not, though, a precise diagnosis along the narrow lines of orthodox classification—which are anyway today disintegrating—is not possible. It is seen increasingly that such classifications do not correspond to the reality of observed fact and are much too restrictive. In practice, the doctor is frequently confronted by a patient who presents no organic complaint: in such a case the patient does not *have* an illness, he *is ill*. What can one do?

This is one of the most important questions for the young general practitioner. Every day he encounters patients whose cases he does not understand, for they do not in any way correspond with those he saw in hospital as a student. He hasn't been trained to deal with such patients. Forced to confine himself to strict schemata which are dinned into him—little realising when he starts work, that there may be patients 'different' from those which he has been shown—he searches desperately for a recognised illness, ordering laboratory tests and useless X-rays. If, after such systematic investigation, he is unable to put a name to the illness, the patient is classed as suffering from a 'functional', if not imaginary or hypochondriac condition. For those who will not 'play the game' of illness as taught there is no choice other than to forego therapy—always hard to countenance, both for the patient and for the doctor (can one ever be sure that one has not made a mistake?)—or the prescription of some all-embracing and heavy-handed treatment, poorly tolerated because it is not really required, and which creates more problems than it cures.

It would be absurd to debate the real value of such drastic treatments in the serious cases where they are required: they are responsible for medicine's greatest successes today. Our aim is to draw attention to the fact that these forms of treatment are useless for the majority of cases seen by the general practitioner; in use, all they do is create side-effects.

Homoeopathic Treatment

The homoeopathic doctor who is fully cognisant of the meaning of the law of similars and thoroughly familiar with the *Homoepathic Materia Medica* can approach therapy quite differently. His knowledge of the *materia medica* gives him access to an extremely wide range of distinct therapeutic treatments for complaints of all sorts, from a straightforward injury to a functional disorder. As soon as he recognises an analogy between the patient's clinical picture and one of those described in the *materia medica* he discovers, as it were, a prescription for a homoeopathic remedy. This is made, so to speak, 'in direct contact' with the clinical syndrome. All one has to do is compare the patient's syndrome with one set in motion in a healthy person by a toxic substance. Described in the same terms, and established according to the same criteria, the two are easily comparable.

The significance of the symptoms noted during the observation phase is twofold: they are signs of an illness (meaning, in general terms, a disorder); and equally they denote a medicament whose action is analogous.

Through his double training (clinical training on the one hand, homoeopathic training on the other) the homoeopath has two systems by means of which he can interpret the patient's symptoms. There is the classical system, which he learned and used during his training and to which he should always turn first, so as to establish a fixed diagnosis whenever that is possible. There is also the homoeopathic system, which he has learned to use by studying the *materia medica* and the law of similars. He should use this latter secondarily, to decide whether or not the patient might be treated homoeopathically.

In certain clearly defined cases (infrequent in everyday practice), a straightforward diagnosis can be made and orthodox treatment is called for. No one would consider treating cerebrospinal meningitis, typhoid or a myocardial infarctus homoeopathically.

Most frequently the patient has a recognised disease (bronchits, measles, angina, cystitis, an allergy syndrome), or a 'functional' complaint (such as dysmenorrhoea) or a psychosomatic illness (spasmodic colitis, migraine, etc.). Orthodox therapy in these cases is often deceptive: it may cope with the symptom which is causing most bother but usually it does so only for a limited time, and very often the same symptom or one very like it reappears.

Homoeopathic treatment, on the other hand, is much easier to carry out and, in our opinion, often more effective. It allows one to treat with equal success readily identified diseases such as measles, angina and otitis, and less clearcut illnesses such as asthma or eczema, in which a person's individual reaction is very much more important.

The remedy to be prescribed for each observed clinical case is that which, in experiment, has displayed a pattern of symptoms similar to those observed in the patient. Once the analogy has been established, the medicament is prescribed in a minute reactive dose. These infinitesimal doses, tolerated by patients of all ages, are devoid of toxicity and possess absolutely no side-effects—something which cannot be said for most orthodox medicines.

They are indeed *reactive* doses: a healthy person can take them without effect. They work only in a person who has already been sensitised by an illness. This might seem odd, but it has been observed countless times in clinical practice, as well as in experiments with animals. (In the latter case, the effect of a homoeopathic remedy prescribed in an infinitesimal dilution can show up only after the animal has been sensitised by an artificially induced illness.)

We think it is important to underline this characteristic at a time when, in many different circles, there is talk of the increasing toxicity of certain drugs and when approximately a third of all medical conventions in the world are devoted to iatrogenic (doctor-created) illnesses and to accidents during treatment.

The homoeopathic doctor's consultation, then, comprises several successive phases, proceeding from listening and observation to the therapeutic prescription best suited to the individual patient. Homoeopathic therapy depends on a precise technique using the law of similars as an artbiter between the patient's clinical picture and the clinical picture as described in the *materia medica*. It is categorically not in opposition to orthodox treatment—quite the reverse, it complements it. The homoeopath does not contest either the action or the worth of classical methods and medicaments: they are undeniably useful in treating a number of clearly defined illnesses. He differs from his colleagues only in his willingness to have systematic recourse to the law of similars whenever that law may be applied.

LITTLE KNOWN SCIENTIFIC FACTS

Although it is often considered as a purely theoretical process, homoeopathic therapy is actually based firmly on experiment. Only after experimenting on himself and his pupils for many years did Hahnemann define the rules which are the foundation of homoeopathic practice: the law of similars (subsequently admitted as a general law) and the habitual use of infinitesimal doses. In general biological terms the law of similars has been accepted, without too much difficulty, as being applicable at least in certain areas, although not as a universal law governing all medical phenomena. The habitual and systemic use of infinitesimal doses, on the other hand, has always been criticised and doubt has therefore cast on their effect. Yet, for more than a hundred and fifty years, homoeopaths the world over have used homoeopathic remedies with great success. But criticism has persisted, for it has been hard to concede that medicaments prescribed in such minute doses could have the least effect.

Until recently, homoeopathic cures—duly described to scientific gatherings or published in specialist reviews—were immediately treated as suspect. It was said that they were obtained through the power of suggestion, the *belief* of the patient in homoeopathic treatment alone being sufficient. People even went so far as to liken such treatment to the magic cures achieved by shamans and sorcerers! They insinuated also, with a wry smile, that nature was responsible for a lot, that the cure was spontaneous, and that in all cases homoeopathic remedies played no part, acting merely as common placebos.

These systematic, ritual criticisms of homoeopathy, as tedious as they were unnecessary, ultimately became almost amusing, because they displayed such a total misunderstanding of what homoeopathy is all about. The detractors failed to realise that homoeopaths *themselves* first had the idea of using the placebo method, so as to have better control over the *real* effects of the remedies they were prescribing. Hahnemann, unknown to the experimental 'guinea-pig', often ordered the use of pillules of a neutral substance instead of pillules impregnated with the medicinal substance which he was studying. Bellows perfected this method, and as early as 1906 carried out an experiment on *Belladonna* in the United States using an experimental 'control'.

According to the scientific norms today prevailing, the only facts which can be considered as having objective validity are those which can be measured and reproduced under identical experimental conditions, and those which arise from statistical studies.

Clearly such rules are highly restricting, and in no way correspond to the spirit of homoeopathy nor to the temperament of homoeopathic doctors, who are more used to researching the individual characteristics of each patient than to classifying into set pigeon-holes, subjects who show identical reactions to the same type of attack. However, such a step can be taken, on condition that the field of study is clearly defined.

Similarly, some years ago it seemed neither necessary nor useful for the development of homoeopathy to carry out animal experiments. Hahnemann always advocated experiments on humans, rejecting those carried out on animals because he felt that they were too crude and were useless in assisting the doctor in his knowledge of the human organism's sensitivity of reaction to the remedy. 'A dog is unaffected by an ounce of the fresh leaves, flowers and seeds of aconite; what man would not be killed?'

It is one of the scientific contradictions of our time that the establishment demands animal experiment while at the same time insisting that there can be no extrapolation from animal to Man, on the basis that their reaction pattern and sensitivity are quite different.

We have ourselves often been involuntary victims of this intellectual vicious circle. What response did we get when we presented our observations?—that they held no value because they were isolated. When, later, we carried out trials on animals which gave rise to statistical studies and which produced objective, reproducible proof, the reply was still that this proved nothing: no conclusion about animals could be related to Man. In spite of these contradictions we continued patiently with our exhaustive experiments and discussions, convinced that in the long run a real dialogue without *a priori* conditions would be instituted.

In spite of the scepticism of classical medicine and of some members of the homoeopathic fraternity (who only added to the numerous technical difficulties inherent in our proceedings), pharmacologists have for some years been able to carry out laboratory trials on animals using the classical experimental rules and hence with the necessary safeguards.

One has to remember two essentials: homoeopathic medicines are used in quantities so tiny that they are not measurable by the normal techniques. But a biological reaction (that of a cell, for instance) can give an indirect indication of the medicines effect. Secondly, the homoeopathic medicament has no effect on healthy men and animals. Its action is manifested only in the sensitised animal—hence the special experimental conditions: the animal is deliberately either infected or poisoned beforehand so that it becomes sensitive to the influence of infinitesimal doses which would have no apparent effect on the healthy animal.

An initial series of experiments enabled researchers to demonstrate the specific detoxifying effect of infinitesimal doses.

The first in both time and importance—indeed, it was a genuine innovation—was carried out in Strasbourg by Mlle L. Warmser on behalf of Father Lapp. Mlle Warmser is now a member of the French Academy of Pharmacy. The procedure used is, superficially, extremely simple. It consists of poisoning an animal and then studying the manifestations of the toxicosis as it develops. Subsequently, one observes the effects of injecting the same toxic substance in various dilutions.

Arsenic poisoning is well known. When an animal (a rat in this case) is poisoned by a strong but not lethal dose of arsenic, part of the toxicity (some 35%) is quickly eliminated (in about $1\frac{1}{2}$ hours) by urination. At the end of this period there is no longer any trace of arsenic in the urine: the poison has established itself in various of the experimental animal's tissues.

At varying times after they had been poisoned, different groups of animals were injected with minute doses of arsenic. Each time, there was renewed elimination of arsenic in the urine, even though natural elimination had ceased several weeks previously.

The experiment was reproducible and gave constant results. Experiments using other toxic substances produced similar results.

These results were a first stage in gaining credibility for the theory of the minimum dose. The next stage was to study the effect of such doses on animal diseases which resembled human diseases as closely as possible. J. Bildet carried out a particularly successful illustrative experiment in Bordeaux, later writen up as a thesis and articles.

Carbon tetrachloride poisoning induces experimental hepatitis, defined as much by its evolution as by the lesion and biological syndrome it triggers, is habitually used to study the action of different medicaments.

Homoeopathic doctors currently use phosphorus in treating viral hepatitis. It was, therefore, of even greater interest to study the possible action of dilutions of white phosphorus on hepatitis in the rat, because the anatamopathological lesions and the biological syndromes triggered by the two sorts of

93

poisoning are very similar, and so this fact allowed verification at the same time of the law of similars.

It was carried out on 150 rats divided into three groups: a control, some poisoned, and some treated (one group treated by dilutions of phosphorus 7c, one group by dilutions of phosphorus 15c after poisoning). The experiment provided objective evidence, through biological examination, of the curative effects of dilutions of phosphorus (Phosphorus 7c and Phosphorus 15c) on toxic hepatitis in rats caused by carbon tetrachloride. The evidence was just as good using anatamopathological examination by optical and electron microscopes.

A toxic dose of phosphorus can lead to hepatitis, and this can be measured objectively by changes in the function of the liver. An infinitesimal, nontoxic dose of the same substance can be used, as we might expect, to treat hepatitis, which has exactly the same symptoms.

This is an excellent experiment in as much as it demonstrated the pharmacological activity of minute doses and the potential importance of the law of similars in choosing a therapy. It also drew attention to a number of facts which were well known to homoeopaths but not to those doing classical medical research. For instance, the infinitesimal dilutions of phosphorus which act on an animal with carbon tetrachloride poisoning apparently have no effect on a healthy animal. For three months, groups of rats were given a daily injection of phosphorus, one group in a dilution of 7c, the other 15c. Examination showed that in none of them was there any detectable change in the cell structure or any measurable biological modification.

Yet these apparently inactive dilutions have a real protective effect, as J. Bildet was able to demonstrate in a second series of experiments. The rats were divided into three uniform groups: a control group which was injected with a physiological serum; a second group injected with phosphorus 7c, and a third group injected with phosphorus 15c. After injection, all were poisoned with carbon tetrachloride.

Before poisoning no change was observable in any group. On poisoning, only those which had received the simple physiological serum injection showed the expected symptoms of toxic hepatitis. The rats in the other two groups developed only a benign and short-lived form of hepatitis; it appeared that they had been protected by the phosphorus dilutions.

This curious fact had already been observed by other workers in other laboratories. With the help of H. Colas we ourselves were able to demonstrate it, very neatly, using cultured cells.

The lymphoblast transformation test is currently used to study a variety of immune reactions: in the presence of certain substances of vegetable origin called lectins (or *phytohaemaglutinins*), a lymphocyte changes into a lymphoblast. The ways and means of this transformation are well known and understood. One of these lectins, *Phytolacca americana*, or pockweed, is often used by homoeopathic doctors in an infinitesimal dilution for a variety of conditions, especially angina, rheumatism and infectious mononeucleosis. We thought it would be interesting to try to find out whether this substance which, in a large dose, can trigger the mitogenesis of a lymphocyte in culture—that is to say, transform a lymphocyte into a lymphoblast—could, on the other hand, block the reaction if used in an infinitesimal dose.

The experiment was carried out at Montpellier. It showed that, while a weighable dose of *Phytolacca* effectively caused the lymphoblastic transformation, an infinitesimal dose had no apparent effect on a normal lymphocyte, whatever dilution (5c, 7c, 9c, 15c) was used. On the other hand, if the lymphocytes were put for 15 minutes in tubes containing dilutions of 5c, 7c, 9c or 15c of *Phytolacca*, they became impervious to the action of other lectins (PHA in this case), and the lymphoblastic transformation no longer took place—or, at the least, was considerably retarded.

This experiment of ours further demonstrated the effect of infinitesimal dilutions and the value of the law of similars. A substance well known to immunologists as causing, at certain concentrations, mitogenesis of a cultured lymphocyte, at extremely low concentrations blocked that very same mitogenesis.

This opens an important area for pharmacological research. The action of medicinal substances is normally known, studied or utilised only within a certain target band, limited at the top end by the toxicity of the substance being studied and at the lower end by its lack of effect. But this apparent lack of effect is only because the action does not conform to the measuring methods currently in use. By modifying such methods one could discover different properties for every known substance! It is these which homoeopaths have always observed in clinical and therapeutic practice. This aspect should be explored by current investigatory practice, so that a *pharmacology of the infinitesimal* may be created. It is our contention that such a step would be of extreme interest for the future of medicine.

Laboratory experiments allow us to demonstrate and measure the very real effect of infinitesimal doses of medicines in general use amongst homoeopathic doctors. But there remains another type of experiment which must be carried out if the demonstration is to be complete: the statistical study of Man.

Professor J. Bernard recently wrote: 'It would be interesting to know and compare the action of homoeopathic remedies and placebos—it is amazing that this simple test has not been tried.' There are two major reasons for this. Firstly, the special conditions in which homoeopathic doctors usually work—for an exclusively private clientele, looking for the particular (each patient's individual reaction) rather than the general (an artificially defined stereotyped syndrome). Secondly, the lack of interest in carrying out such trials shown by universities and teaching hospitals.

The experiment *can* successfully be carried out if the reactionary syndrome isolated is sufficiently clearly defined in its manifestations and development, and if a homoeopathic remedy able to trigger an analagous syndrome is used.

A study of the action of dilutions of phosphorus on viral hepatitis would seem an ideal example. The experiment was suggested to some researchers who wanted to write a thesis on the subject, but no specialist faculty has so far accepted the project. Yet J. Bildet's experiment clearly demonstrates the therapeutic value of dilutions of phosphorus in toxic hepatitis in rats. In addition, no effective treatment is known for viral hepatitis—the objection is made that it cures itself. If this is true, the cure usually does not come about except after a great deal of trouble.

In practice, one can very well study a group of fifty patients treated with phosphorus and compare them with fifty untreated patients to see if there is not an objective statistical difference, using as points of reference the subjective symptoms (asthenia, nausea) and the objective symptoms (transaminase, bilirubinaemia, etc.), all the while observing the time it takes the two groups to return to normal.

The work will undoubtedly be done one day, for the dialogue between homoeopathy and orthodox medical teaching is becoming more amicable all the time. But homoeopaths must, if they wish to be understood by the medical faculties, resist the temptation to arm themselves with a dogma. Instead, they should realise that they have a method which can push back the boundaries of therapy. There is a growing awareness that, while the field of available action is limited, it is of great value. Professor Hamburger has described it as 'the spearhead of medicine'.

We saw a recent example in a highly technological surgical department. In spite of extremely sophisticated equipment, the incidence of pre- and post-operatory pulmonary obstruction remained very high. A female student in the department, knowing the manifestations of antimony poisoning (which correspond completely with the symptoms displayed by her patients) suggested giving them treatment supplementary to the classical therapy. She suggested a dilution of antimony, something which homoeopaths have traditionally used for certain types of bronchitis with pulmonary obstruction. The condition of the twenty patients so treated compared extremely favourably in its development with that of the regular patients treated solely by classical means.

There are many other possible experiments of this type, either to confirm the action of a homoeopathic remedy in general use amongst homoeopathic doctors, or to find new means of therapy for certain syndromes for which there is currently no treatment. For this to be brought about, homoeo-pathy must be recognised as a viable means of treating certain illnesses or certain kinds of patients, and not be rejected out of hand as a result of simplistic partisanship.

In addition, the experimental method which Hahnemann defined and put into practice at the end of the 18th century must finally be given proper consideration, so that the field of scientific enquiry is widened to include hitherto-unexplored territory.

We have given some examples, provided some proofs, and drawn some conclusions from experience; nevertheless, we have passed over many other curious facts which deserve attention. We hope the examples we have given will not be treated solely as proofs to rebut the antagonistic but rather that they will provoke thought and questioning.

The results obtained over a number of years raise more questions than they answer. The remedies work, yes, but *how* do they work? At what level does this action take place? What is the stereochemical structure of the molecules in the great dilutions in which the remedies are used? How are they carried into the body? Why do they become active so rapidly? Why does the medicinal action vary according to the concentration when apparently there has been no change in the chemical constitution? Why is their effect seen only in a sensitive organ or cell, with no apparent effect on the healthy version? How can mercury be used to treat angina, even if used at a lesser concentration than is found in atmospheric pollution? How can silica, which in a measurable dose is known to be inactive, become in a minimal dose an extremely useful medicine in the teatment of chronically festering wounds? How can sodium chloride, common salt, become a thoroughly effective remedy when used in dilution?

So many questions! We are sure that in the end they will arouse the curiosity and imagination of researchers and lead to the development of fundamental research which will reveal homoeopathy in its true light.

CHAPTER IV

Rumours

Homoeopathy is still surrounded by a multitude of myths and rumours. We would like to devote this chapter to rebutting such current notions, for accusations and reservations arise most often from a misunderstanding of the facts.

Having studied the basis of homoeopathy as a therapeutic technique and as a medical theory which happily complements the orthodox approach to the patient and the disease, the next step is to remove the mystery from it, to emphasis its practical aspects and to show that it is neither mysterious nor out-of-date, neither long nor complicated and that its efficacy has been proved.

IT IS MYSTERIOUS

What is a homoeopathic medicine? How is it prepared? What techniques are used?

The fact is that each medicine owes its individuality and its uniqueness to the way in which it is pharmaceutically prepared. This method of preparation has been laid down since 1965 in the French pharmaceutical codex. Here is the official wording:

In the 1965 codex, in the monograph *Homoeopathic Preparations*, the method of dilution is described in the following manner (page 1350):

99

Preparation

(a) Centesimal Dilutions

Take new flasks and corks, washed in water and dried, the number of which should correspond to the required number of centesimal dilutions. In the first flask place one part (by weight) of the basic substance; dilute it one hundred times by means of the appropriate diluent, and shake at least one hundred times. The dilution so obtained is designated one c.

Take one part (by volume) of this 1c pour it into the second flask, which should already contain ninety-nine parts of the diluent; shake one hundred times as before. The dilution so obtained is designated 2c. Proceed in the same manner until the required dilution is reached.

(b) Decimal dilutions

Proceed in a similar manner, but for 'hundredths' read 'tenths'.

(c) Decimal or centesimal triturations

Take the active solid substance, which you have previously reduced to a fine powder, and triturate it carefully for a long time in a mortar with a small amount of the lactose being used as the medium. Continue the trituration adding, little by little, the rest of the lactose. The respective quantities of the active substance and the lactose are calculated so as to obtain the first decimal or centesimal trituration. Take one part of this trituration and triturate it as before with nine or ninety-nine parts of lactose in order to obtain (respectively) the second decimal or the second centesimal trituration. Proceed in the same manner in order to obtain the third decimal and the third centesimal trituration. After this, switch to a liquid diluent and contine as given above for dilutions.

Preparation of the Medicine

'Hahnemann technique' (separate flasks)

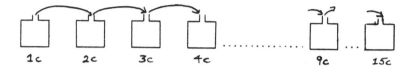

1c   2c   3c   4c   9c   15c

Dilution to 1/100
Vigorous succussion, or 'potentisation'
c9 = ninth centesimal Hahnemann dilution

Dilution to 1/10
Vigorous succussion, or 'potentisation'
d3 (or 3x) = third decimal Hahnemann dilution

- *The number indicates the degree of the dilution*
- *The letters (c, d) indicate the technique of preparation*
- The term 'potentisation', often used in place of 'succussion', introduces a philosophic idea which has no place in the experimental domain

---

As you see, there is nothing mysterious in all this. The bottle of pills in your pocket represents a medicine prepared in the laboratory by a particular technique, subject to precise and clearly stated controls. This medicine has a known pharmacological action which can be demonstrated and experimentally reproduced. It must contain 'something', otherwise there would be no cap on the bottle! You do not 'believe' in aspirin or penicillin: these medicines exist and you have confidence in them. Similarly, you do not have to 'believe' in *Nux vomica*

101

c5 or phosphorus c15: these medicines exist and you may have confidence in them too. Their action has been demonstrated. The reasoning behind their prescription has been verified by experiments on animals and plants.

Homoeopathic medicines, like the other medicines to which you are accustomed, do not have a 100% success-rate in every case. Their prescription and their effectiveness both depend upon the circumstances, your doctor's knowledge and your individual reaction to the substance. *Their therapeutic action depends entirely on the dosage.* Sometimes you will need a strong dose of the medicine to treat a certain condition; sometimes a weaker dose will be needed. Often an infinitesimal dose will be necessary to help your reaction.

There is no sense, then, in distinguishing between 'hard' and 'soft' medicine. It is all a question of choice in the means of treatment and in the adaptation of these means, and in the quantities of the remedies prescribed.

To sum up: the doctor must be 'reformed' in order to recover his true role of healer. When one uses a homoeopathic remedy one is using something more than 'sugared water'. It is a medicine like any other and its character is determined by its method of preparation.

Whether a medicine is of mineral, vegetable or animal origin, its origins can always be traced. Thus you can trace this bottle of *Belladonna* 5c, from which you have just taken three pills for your sore throat, right back to its origins. The berries and leaves of this *Belladonna* plant were picked at such-and-such an hour of such-and-such a day in such-and-such a season. Even the name and address of the person who picked them are known: he or she belonged to a certain part of the country and was well versed in its flora. The subsequent history of the plant is fully recorded: maceration, filtration, dilution, succussion, and its incorporation into the pillules. At each stage of these operations, renewed tests of quality and identification are carried out in accordance with techniques which are officially laid down. The base of the medicine, whether in pillule or in globule form, is lactose, a sugar selected because its porosity is such that it is impregnated regularly and homogenously by the medicinal substance. Special turbines work for forth-eight hours to turn out this pillule, which started as a crystal of lactose—rather in the same way that an oyster naturally builds up its pearl. When the substances are of mineral origin—phosphorus, sulphur, arsenic, sodium chloride or mercury—the same precautions are taken as if the substances are of animal origin—snake and bee venom, or cuttlefish ink—whose family, species and chemical make-up are known. You can see, then, that there is nothing mysterious about the preparation of a medicine.

The Instability of the Pills

What about their supposed instability? They must not be touched by hand ... avoid peppermint, coffee etc ... Oh! all the fine stories! They are all figments of the imagination and of the credulity of generations of doctors and patients, who can produce no vestige of proof to support their assertions. Without entering into fruitless argument (for myths must be respected for what they are), here is what can be asserted as a result of experiments on animals and of daily observation. Experiments using a given substance (*Apis*: bee) carried out on guinea-pigs were repeated, making the animals take peppermint syrup and peppermint leaves. The results were just the same with or without the peppermint. So what? We know that many patients do indeed eat peppermints during their treatment—especially children—and the remedies work just the same!

Thanks to improved techniques, it has recently become possible to observe the structure of the pills. Photographs taken with an electronic microscope have shown that the pills are composed of concentric layers intersected by fine micropores. Chromatography has shown that, as one would logically expect with such a structure, the substance penetrates right to the centre of the pill. It seems that the argument against touching the pill, because it was supposed to be unstable, because the active agent was assumed to be confined to the surface regions, has now been exploded.

IT IS OUT OF DATE

A rumour is born, it spreads, it grows, it feeds on itself and it ends up by hiding the plain truth. The most important thing to do is *not to confuse homoeopathy with the homoeopath*. The homoeopath is a doctor, or sometimes a quack, who prescribes remedies with Latin names followed by a number: 5c, 15c ...

He is a person with his full share of preconceptions—to many he is an eccentric, an exponent of fringe medicine. Some homoeopaths encourage this image, which protects them from having to answer major questions.

We have all of us met doctors who surround themselves with an aura of mystery and seem to have 'secret knowledge', which cannot be 'revealed' either to the patient or to any pupils they may have ... If it is not a mystery, why is it not taught at medical school? Why can 'healers' or anyone else get the relevant medicines without a prescription? Why do some homoeopaths dispense their medicines themselves, and give them to their patients direct? Why do they send abroad for certain 'special' dilutions?

Here is a body of questions which patients are entitled to ask. In order to answer them, and to show that homoeopathy is neither an old-fashioned idea nor an anti-scientific technique, it is necessary for doctors to have the opportunity of learning about it. This, however, entails a fundamental change in the way medicine is taught.

A Doctor Must Become a 'Healer' Again

The current problem of medical education has been put clearly in the writings of Dr Escause and Dr Sournia. This education has become so technical that we have got to the stage of forgetting that the diseased organ, together with its biological or cellular changes, are actually part of a human being. So our concern must be to ensure that, while the organic side of disease, its quantitative aspect, is not neglected, this should be seen in conjunction with its qualitative aspect. 'Since 1968 the universities have been turning out learned doctors who are ill prepared for what society expects of them … Medicine which makes machines and numbers take precedence over people is a bad kind of medicine [Sournia: *Ces malades qu'on fabrique* p. 229].' Indeed, all studies of stress show the intricate connection between physical and mental illness, and bear witness to the fundamental importance of the reaction of the individual patient to his illness.

Students of medicine have, little by little, lost sight of this qualitative aspect, although a certain number of them—the 'real doctors'—are strongly aware of it. Their questions, echoed by their patients, have raised the issue, and today's medical fraternity must provide some answers. This social phenomenon is only a few years old, and is akin to the ecological movement (which has lately become a force in politics). We must take firm note of it in order to understand fully its blessings and its curses.

In order to give medical technology its rightful place (which, however important it may be, is not always the first place), it is essential to use orthodox symptomatology—i.e., to study the signs of illness, so as to be able to make or direct a diagnosis, by means of the senses: sight (objective signs), hearing (interrogation, sounding by stethoscope), touch (palpation), smell (secretions).

Having had the professional satisfaction of establishing a diagnosis—or, rather, to have made it without the help of any instrument—you are in a position to know what 'supplementary' or radiological examinations will be essential in the interests of the patient, not only taking into account his clinical history but seeing him in his social context.

For instance, there would be no point in calling for immediate surgery in a case which could, under supervision, be left for several months, if such surgery would lead to any family or professional conflict which might have serious consequences for the future of the patient. Similarly, it would be senseless to carry out certain examinations, costly for society and dangerous for the patient, if there were no way that they could lead to the prescription of a more effective therapy than could be undertaken without them. Here human factors, connected with the personality of the doctor himself, come into play: in addition to his technical medical knowledge, he should have also an appreciation of the social situation.

The 'False Sick', or How to Die Cured!

The study of homoeopathy depends above all on orthodox symptomatology. It is, therefore, inconceivable that one should learn homoeopathy or practise it except on this essential basis; it even seems to us necessary that symptomatology should be included as one of the subjects to be studied in a homoeopathy course, since it is through this main clinical means that real homoeopathic symptomatology—that is, the study of the most characteristic signs of the sufferer—may be carried out. Homoeopathic symptomatology is not opposed to orthodox symptomatology; it complements it, giving it exactly that dimension which is found in current practice.

Let us not forget that a medical student should be trained for what he is going to find in everyday life, and not in order that he may discover once a year the famous syndrome of such and such a professor, who has given his name to a disease of which only fifty-two cases are known to have occurred in the whole world.

What is the student going to find? Difficulties in coping with life, physical symptoms which reveal the reactions of patients to conflict—but he does not yet know that these clinical pictures correspond, in therapeutic terms, to homoeopathic remedies. This fact makes it imperative that homoeopathy should be taught at medical school as a technique among other therapeutic techniques, since it can be an answer to the requirements of 80% of so-called 'functional' patients, who are in reality in the process of creating their own organic ill-nesses.

In this way, homoeopathy can enable a student to be no longer helpless when faced with so-called 'unclassifiable' patients; for there is at the present time a gap in medical treatment which leads doctors to reject 'nervous psychosomatics, patients bringing long lists of their symptoms, and hypochondriacs, who together make up three-quarters of those coming to the consulting-room. [Escande: *Les Malades* p. 173]'.

Homoeopathy can provide the answer for 'those "false patients" who are neither cured nor comforted by desperate medical measures' (Escande again). Such an appreciation of the problem by one of the best modern educationalist arouses simultaneously our irritation and our interest: irritation, because there cannot be any such thing as 'false' patients; interest, because we are able to suggest a logical and comprehensive solution.

The first step, then, has to concern therapeutic efficacy. Any interpretation which one may subsequently make of the results of such therapy or the mechanism by which works it is a personal question, and irrelevant to the practice of homoeopathy. We did not need to ponder on the vital processes to prescribe china-clay for nose-bleeding or *Gelsemium* for panic; on the other hand, it was possible to take further therapeutic measures by studying the case as a whole and treating the deep-rooted causes of these complaints (which in one case, after verification that there was no local cause, proved to be the troubles of adolescence and, in the other, difficulty in fitting into society). This meant that the doctor/patient relationship was deepened without prior assumption. Another advantage is that this study of a therapy is not subject to the dictates of fashion or to the caprice of the drug-houses. Homoeopathic remedies have been prepared and prescribed according to the same techniques for more than one hundred and fifty years.

Research is constantly putting us on our guard against the appearance of resistant strains of microbes and viruses and forecasting new virus epidemics against which we will have little in the way of therapeutic resources. Here again we are reassured by homoeopathy, which is unchanging in its principles and its practice, since it makes use of a weapon which is itself unchanging: the normal reaction of the individual.

'The Workman Makes His Tool, Then the Tool Makes the Workman'

Homoeopathy could be a means of reconciling technical

symptomatology and the symptomatology of the individual. Moreover, it is wrong to think that homoeopathy is difficult to learn and that twenty-five years' experience is necessary in order to practice it. *Experience,* apart from the time factor which alone can make one aware of the relatively of events, is valuable through the intensity of the action one undertakes and the constructive criticism which one associates with it. Making the same mistakes over and over again gives the wrong kind of experience. The only way to make progress is to keep on questioning what you are learning and teaching, provided you have a solid foundation which can stand up to this questioning.

That is what we are trying to do in our teaching, which consists more in *teaching how to learn* than in passing on cut-and-dried knowledge. The workman has to make his tool; after that, it is the tool which makes the workman.

Without any doubt, it is within the range of every medical student who wishes to specialise to learn homoeopathy. It is a question of technique. As always, there will be some who will quickly understand it well and others who, as in every other field, will drag their feet.

It is not a question of reducing homoeopathy to a simplistic technique and a set of standard prescriptions, but one of giving it its due place: that of a truly experimental science, with a part to play in contemporary medical thought.

This necessity to teach homoeopathy corresponds today to a general demand: from doctors, both GPs and specialists, increasingly from medical students, and from patients and health authorities.

It seems to us essential that homoeopathy should be studied at medical school as a therapeutic method which is permanently open to criticism, since it has the advantage of being an open system based on great clinical experinece.

There is a flagrant disparity between its effectiveness and the lack of serious literature on the subject; and this should give rise to many questions and investigations from which homoeopathy would emerge unharmed because, in spite of considerable errors of interpretation, it undoubtedly possesses the answers to many health problems.

Finally, and this is no mean advantage, such an approach would counter the stupid claim that it is 'anti-medicine'!

IT IS ONLY FOR 'WELL' PEOPLE

Homoeopathy—that's for 'people who have nothing the matter with them', for 'nervous people', for 'women with headaches' ... and what about men?

You hear such remarks a hundred times over, and they deserve attention: it is worth trying to see how they come about.

An illness does not develop in a week. It is the result of the malfunction of organs. All the time, your body is continually destroying and rebuilding itself. Precise and delicate mechanisms seek to maintain a dynamic equilibrium between the phenomena of destruction and construction. The body spends its time adapting by finding a new equilibrium after a physical or psychological disturbance. When these mechanisms are going out of order, when the machine is running out of steam—*that* is the time to act. It is for this reason that we think homoeopathy is one of the best ways of carrying out preventative medicine at this stage; and this is why:

Real Preventative Medicine
Preventative medicine today consists mainly of systematically tracking down a number of diseases—a point in its favour, especially in the cases of tuberculosis, diabetes and hypercholesorol situations—but also of carrying out **medical check-ups** which, to date, do not seem to have had any practical result in the prevention of disease, in either a social or an economic context.

Medical examinations applied to a certain section of the population would be justified if, after a number of years, the section examined regularly when well, was in better health than another section which had not been so examined, or if the amount paid out by medical insurance was less than had been anticipated. *Up to now there has been no proof of this!* [Our italics]. (Sournia, p. 138.)

On the other hand, it is necessary to regard prevention in its own context, which is not always exclusively medical. For example, in 1973 in France, 70.7% of the deaths of young people between the ages of 15 and 24 were due to traffic accidents. At this stage, then, prevention should be more educational than medical. The money used should not be invested in the same place, although we know that accidents which are really camouflaged 'suicides' are not the prerogative of the young, but may also be due to drivers full of tranquillisers having had a few glasses of alcohol—a situation for which France, unhappily, holds the record.

Mortality Among Young People in France
Per 1,000, Died Between the Ages of 15 and 24 (Year: 1973)

Accidents	70.7%
Tumours	6.7%
Cardio-vascular diseases	3.3%
Digestive troubles	1.6%

Source: INSEE Almost all of the accidents are road accidents.

A study of the official statistics of the causes of death or disablement shows how difficult it is to separate the different causes of morbidity. An observer accustomed to synthesising would know at what level it would be artificial, although perhaps necessary, to make a separate count of cardiovascular or respiratory ailments or premature senility, knowing the great number of aetiological factors involved in these ailments, notably tobacco and alcohol poisoning. Here, again, it is a question of the way the individual behaves with regard to his health.

It appears, indeed, that the patients who call for these medical examinations are, in the main, content with the figures quoted for the results, but that these have no effect at all on their behaviour towards their own health.

On the other hand, there is no therapy, apart from advice on hygiene, which is applicable to the stage of illness below the clinical level; that is to say when, although a lesion is already present, there are as yet no exterior signs nor anything to register in a biological examination.

'The Functional is Organic'

What can one say in this case? A lesion is most often established gradually and the functional disorder will appear to have no cause, since 'a functional disorder is organic' (cf. Klotz: *Revue de medicine fonctionelle*. April, 1973). Indeed, even if it is not possible in present technical conditions to identify a lesion in its initial stages, there will always be a molecular, biochemical or vaso-motor disturbance at the level of the malfunctioning cells. The problem of knowing whether the functional disorder precedes the organic disorder, the lesion, or whether it comes after it, will probably never be solved and, indeed, loses much of its importance in our particular approach. This is because we do not have to interpret the patient's symptoms but to convert them, often very early on, into signs which indicate a certain homoeopathic remedy in the given clinical situation—and, moreover, at a stage when there are no other means of therapeutic section.

It is, then, a question of true preventative medicine since, through our *knowledge of the individual reaction of the patient to his illness,* we have the means (dependent on various aetiological circumstances) of acting on a person of a given type of sensitivity and with a particular known morbid predisposition.

Knowing in Advance How to Direct Preventative Medicine to Everyone's Advantage

Similarly, we can employ the most sophisticated techniques to track down disease on those groups of subjects whom we know to be predisposed towards contracting certain diseases. For example, for a sulphur type we would direct our attention towards discovering signs of incipient diabetes, since he would be predisposed to such a pathological development.

We know classes of people who react to chronic infections, to chemotherapy or to certain vaccinations by producing polyps or warts.

This particular reaction with this type of patient would make us specially vigilant in looking for very early signs of precancerous lesions—in the intestines, for example, since this is a current problem of medicine: it is believed that systematic investigation by rectoscope or by radiology would make it possible to discover a certain number of lesions at a stage before cancer has developed. It is necessary to choose which investigations are carried out, since one always has to strike a balance between the medical value of such an operation and its cost in financial terms. By choosing the groups which are particularly endangered—which we are able to do thanks to our special approach—we can practise true preventative medicine with the maximum value in medical and financial terms.

'Predictive biochemistry' can be one of the fruitful elements of preventive medicine, provided its use is limited to certain 'high spots' of health risk.

Preventive Measures in Homoeopathy

As all modern writings on medicine state repeatedly, the time has come to treat the healthy and not the sick. This would appear to be the most fruitful ground for homoeopathy, provided one can distinguish between what is reversible and what is not, and can know when the prognosis justifies another kind of therapy (chemotherapy or surgery). It is true that there are forms of tuberculosis revealed by X-rays which show no clinical signs of being a condition requiring surgery and which develop without functional involvement, but this evidence implies and justifies the fact that homoeopathy should not be practised except by doctors sufficiently aware of the limits of every method to be able to make an intelligent choice of therapy.

A knowledge of temperaments and of predisposition towards particular diseases also enables us to give people real health education at a very early stage; for *prevention consists of acting at the moment when an individual dearts from his biological rhythm, whenever that may be in his life.* It is easier to maintain an equilibrium than to repair a faulty one. Furthermore, the fact that homoeopathic remedies are not toxic makes it possible to avoid the medication of those in apparently good health. It is a question of teaching people not to spend their time in self-analysis or in 'contemplating their navels' but to distinguish in their particular case between an important symptom and an ordinary, insignificant one.

This does not mean that homoeopathic remedies are ineffective. The greater proportion of all biochemical phenomena occurring in an organism are produced by concentrations in the blood of hormonal substances or prostaglandins in the order of nanograms (one thousand-millionth of a gram) or, in the case of certain neurohormones, of picograms (10^{-12} g). It is, therefore, not a case of a simple placebo effect, even if this is undeniably present in a certain number of cases—as in every other kind of therapy.

Thus, it is at the level of regulating functions that we can act and our attention will be particularly directed, for a certain sort of patient, towards tracking down a certain sort of illness.

This mode of intervention seems to us an obvious one, and yet it has not been applied except in homoeopathic circles. It is an opportunity for our special approach.

Prevention is not possible without information being available at the earliest possible moment; to this end, why should we not make use, as is already being done, of even the medium of children's comics, since prevention is above all a state of mind? Indeed, we must make provision for what medicine will be like in twenty years' time, not on the basis of what it is today but on the basis of what it would have to be as the result of the worldwide evolution of various techniques. This is one of the points which I shall deal with in the section on the attitude of the future.

IT TAKES SO LONG

Does homoeopathy take a long time?

This new attitude towards the prevention of disease has an obvious sociological influence. A new triangular relationship must be established between the patient, the disease and the doctor. After that, because the problems will have been properly stated, it will be possible to select the right therapy in the interest of the patient and of society.

Homoeopathy and Sociology

In the field of health, requirements have changed radically, especially in the industrialised countries with a liberal economy, whereas we continue to respond to them in terms of what they were twenty-five years ago.

As statistics show, the number of patients with organic disease does not grow, but the idea of health has been modified. We note an increase in degenerative cardiovascular diseases and above all in those diseases characterised by depression caused by having to meet difficult situations. This leads, in the terms of H. Pradel, to the creation of a real 'agony market'. The difficulty of adapting to our civilisation produces a disturbance of the normal functioning of an individual, who then looks to medicine to provide the solution; at the present time, though, medicine is not able to take charge of everyone.

> Claiming that we can cure social maladjustment with medicine, or manufacturing drugs and paying out money without achieving the desired goal, treating social anomalies medically with X-rays and tranquilisers; that is the absurd way we behave at the moment.

And further on:

> This use of medication in every difficult situation is not healthy; social conflicts require social remedies, not medicines and X-rays. [Sournia: *Ces malades qu'on fabrique* p. 245.]

It is in such situations that the appeal of the homoeopathic approach is greatest. We are speaking here of the 'hard core' of medical practice, which concerns the health problems of 80% of our current consultations with patients and the therapy which we suggest for them, and is quite divorced from any medical sectarianism concerning other techniques which have proved their worth. In these cases the disease is a variation of the normal health of the individual patient, and the symptoms which he described are alarm signals indicating departure from this norm. Faced with this request for help from a patient who is just becoming ill, the doctor must act as counsellor in suggesting what therapy should be followed; hence the *necessity of knowing the different technical therapies* which can be used in a given clinical situation.

Certainly an ordinary knowledge of human nature or of psychology would lead to the same attitude, but with this difference, which seems an essential one: homoeopathy is able to provide *physical* medical help in the form of the simple remedies it uses, even if the prescribed medicines may appear, whether intentionally or not, like placebos.

There is No Such Thing as an Imaginary Illness

During the long period when an organic disease is gradually building up, there will be weeks, months or even years during which the sick person is not recognised as such by modern orthodox medicine. At best, he will be thought, with a certain false sense of security, to be suffering from a 'functional' disease; at worst, he will be considered as an 'imaginary invalid.', a hypochondriac.

However, there is no such thing as an imaginary invalid. Even before it is possible to make a positive diagnosis of a disease, backed up by supplementary examinations or X-rays, there will still be a clinical disease, which is expressed by symptoms, whose grouping or syndrome requires us to regulate them by a therapy. In this vast field the homoeopathic approach is incomparable.

The Doctor as a Privileged Educationalist

In our opinion, this original approach has several advantages. It avoids the danger of overmedicating the patient at a stage where only minimal or no medication is necessary. It helps him to take charge of himself if he wishes, once he has been informed of what is possible for him in this respect. It allows the doctor to act as a true health counsellor, having regard to the temperament and the potentialities of each of his patients; in this way the doctor avoids being rejected, whether voluntarily or not, by those 'patients' who are most often misunderstood since no appropriate therapy can be suggested for them at the moment. Also, and this we consider most important, it allows the demolition of the barrier between the sick person and the doctor, who is no longer the one who alone wields medical power, but the counsellor, who may be aided by the advice of anyone concerned with providing help. This attitude enables him, while retaining his own position (which is not a higher but a different one), to take decision for the benefit of his patient in full knowledge of the facts.

It is not here a question of conflicts of personality, for no one person can dominate all the fields of medical activity. A hospital attendant specialising in cardiac resuscitation, for example, is technically more competent than many doctors; but it is the doctor, who, after having made a synthesis of all the factors in a case, will make the decision.

Taking personal responsibility for one's own health with the help of people competent in this field; recognising that a patient has the right to know himself and to know why and how he is being treated; being informed of the cost of health within a social group (including the family group)—all these are, to my mind, the main points of contact between the homoeopathic approach and the health problems in present-day society.

Disease Must No Longer Cause Fear

Rather than supply theoretical interpretations of sociological problems, we would prefer to cite concrete cases, typical of those occurring among our patients. Our particular approach leads us to adopt a responsible attitude towards illness, but also more particularly towards health: this includes responsibility towards oneself, but also responsibility towards the way others see the illness (in a family, for example, the children, the grandparents, the husband and wife.)

Little by little the patient reaches the stage where he is no longer afraid of the symptoms, because he sees them as the reaction of his own organism to some exterior cause, a reaction in which *he is going to participate,* since homoeopathy is a reactive therapy in that its aim is to restore normality to an organism influenced by disease.

The M. family is especially typical in this respect. The three children had repeated attacks of nasopharyngitis, accompanied by serious asthmatic bronchitis, which were only slightly helped by antibiotics and corticoids. The mother had disturbed nights, being woken up by those unnerving coughs which parents know so well. Prolonged absences from school were upsetting the children's development. The father was annoyed at seeing his children always ill—and his wife fired from her job, into the bargain—and his temper became worse ... when, that is, he was not able to take refuge from the situation by ignoring it completely.

We were able to practise real health education by teaching the mother to interpret the reactions of her children, and by helping her not to fear the inevitable cold which went on and on, with complications, since with a few homoeopathic medicines, reinforced by the constitutional remedy, it is possible to deal with apparently complicated situations. What is more, this attitude had the advantage of rescuing the children from being 'chronic dependents' and unwilling consumers of useless drugs, use of which should be limited entirely to cases where a patient is no longer able to control his illness simply by stimulating his natural immunity.

There is no need to stress the obvious advantage of avoiding, where possible, a tonsils operation (very frequent among our patients), since no surgical operation is justified unless the indications are that the patient will be in better health after than before it. In practice this is not always the case.

117

Homoeopathy

Mr M., puzzled by seeing the health of his children improved without any psychological influence, since children of three and five are not more susceptible to the magic of antibiotics than to that of *Mercurius solubilis*, comes to us for a consultation. It will be possible, if that is what he wants, to make him aware of his potentialities with respect to his own health, which is becoming unbalanced, and thus to help him to live in accordance with his biological rhythms and his temperament. Of course, we are not able to change his temperament, but we can *help him to use it*.

Mr M. is a choleric type whose condition is aggravated by a sedentary way of life, heavy meals and constant irritations, and he suffers from common digestive troubles, characterised by acidity of the stomach one hour after meals; this is improved by a five-minute siesta. This little picture enables us on the one hand to prescribe the correct homoeopathic remedy to help him but, even more, to explain to him that it is advisable to change his habits. If he does not do so, given a sensitive type like his, it is likely that there will be an accentuation of the spasmodic attacks, which, after years of upset experienced in his digestive tract, may lead to, for example, a gastric ulcer, should there be any inherited predisposition towards one.

From this moment on, Mr M. makes his choice: it is not our place to *impose on him a healthy way of living. But this lifestyle should correspond to the fact that he is himself*, no one else; that is to say, he must take into account his own dynamic, within the context of which the well chosen homoeopathic medicine will act as a regulator.

His sister-in-law, who is labelled a spasmodic type and swallows a whole arsenal of pills without any result, sees her condition improve considerably and become balanced (in imbalance!) through the prescribed remedies. Her children are glad to see that their mother is able to stop being the 'chronic invalid' they have known for eight years and their relationship with her improves markedly.

Homoeopathy's Sociological Importance
Through a patient's requests for advice during a consultation

118

we are able to achieve results which do not involve his overmedication; more difficult is to bring him back to a stage of health and then to maintain it by regular therapy, interspersed with periods when this is no longer necessary.

To a certain number of people, it is possible to explain what are the first signs of biological imbalance in their organism. There is no such thing as an 'imaginary invalid'; the symptoms they feel correspond to *something*. The problem of knowing whether they are the consequence or the cause of molecular malfunction will, perhaps, never be solved; but the homoeopathic approach makes it possible to translate immediately into therapeutic terms the symptoms felt by and observed in the patient.

Let us take the case of an adolescent who is faced with the problem of choosing the right vocational training. He has taken the psychological tests and seen the educational advisers, but his own unexpressed preference lies elsewhere. It is through knowledge of his temperament and of the remedies which have been effectively prescribed for him for quite different reasons that we can find out where his deep-seated interest lies. In this case, it is in horses; and his choice can range anywhere between teaching horse-riding and directing a national stud. The right decision means a well directed and satisfied adolescent.

If the importance of homoeopathy in chronic diseases is obvious, its sociological importance in acute disease is even more apparent. Usually, with our patients, a true case of influenza (Hong Kong epidemic type) lasts only a week, and is not followed by exhaustion or the necessity for tonics or long periods off work. The experience is the same in a certain number of debilitating viral diseases (infectious mononucleosis, viral hepatitis) where it seems, according to clinical tests, that the time spent off work on account of the disease need never exceed three weeks. However, since such statements are based on the experience of current patients, the observed facts are necessarily debatable.

If one is interested in other people—and in the case of a doctor there should be no question about this—then it is easy to play the part of a health educator on various levels, if one knows *how each person can take charge of his own health.* Starting at this level of personal responsibility, some people are able to take a global view of health and their collective responsibility with regard to this problem, and can then try to influence its course. They can take part in study groups or consumer groups, not in order always to criticise what is suggested, but to take part in the decisions which will affect their medical future and that of their children.

HOMOEOPATHY AND COSTS

On the economic level the problem of health is perfectly clear. It is insoluble if things continue in the way they are going at the moment. As Sournia says (p. 23): 'The nation's health used to be a technical problem; it is becoming an economic one. It can no longer be summed up as a fight against microbes or cancer. It affects the financial life of the country.'

The financial scandal of social security grows from year to year. In France, the 'gap' was twenty-four thousand million francs before the health insurance contributions were raised on April 1st, 1979, and this move provided only a temporary improvement. Nowadays, *everyone* is involved, and it is no longer possible to put the burden of responsibility onto other people in order to avoid having to think about one's own responsibility in one's own little world ...

Priorities must be determined and, in order to do this, our attitude towards health and illness must be radically altered. Such an alteration can only come about as the result of joint action by the medical or administrative authorities and by those who are primarily concerned: the patients themselves, determined to tackle these problems once they have been thoroughly acquainted with not only their *rights* but also their *duties*.

Health-economy problems, intricately bound up with a number of complex phenomena, cannot be solved piecemeal but only if seen in a world-wide context. In order to see that this is true, one need only analyse the effect on the economy of medical training as such, of the way doctors' time is wasted, and of the bad use to which both doctors themselves and the hospitals are put.

'The Thyroid and the Computer': A Modern Tale

Medical training can have an effect on the cost of health, as witness the following example, one of dozens which can be found daily: '50% of the thyroid check-ups requested at the Créteil CHU cannot be justified on purely medical grounds.' A paper by Dr Diedisheim states this problem in precise terms:

A computer analysis of the circumstances of 767 examinations showed that nearly 50% of the applications for an examination were more in the nature of 'decoration' than justified on purely medical grounds. The examinations of perfectly normal patients uselessly cluttered up the department of radiotherapy, making it refuse certain urgent cases—the results from which would have been of the greatest importance to this therapy. Furthermore, these examinations involve quite considerable expense if one takes them as a whole: 37 million centimes [about £40,000] could be saved. Each iodine examination costs 704 francs [about £70] each dose of hormones 208 francs [about £20]. The time spent on these examinations adds up to 702 days a year.

To the consideration of expense should be added another result, namely that, no matter what motive these patients had in seeking a consultation, they will be a little more 'set' in their functional syndromes. Indeed, with these patients psychosis and organic disease are closely connected: 98.1% of them have some trauma in their past history; and in 82% of the cases it has been the decisive factor. The trauma is most often psychological; often it is a case of marital or family conflict. The practitioner takes refuge in technology while what people *really* want is a return to the doctor/ patient relationship.

In conclusion, a critical study of thyroid examinations shows that there is a gap in the theoretical and practical

121

training of young doctors. Medicine is no longer an art or a science based on calculable elements, whether concrete or abstract, and ignoring individuality.

On the contrary, a study of the various psychological factors which play a part in the pathology of thyroid diseases shows the extremely *individual* character of the pathology.

We should add that it seems ironical that a computer had to be used, at considerable expense, in order to discover and analyse mistakes in judgment which could have been avoided with a little common sense.

Rights and Duties of the Patient

Another cause of useless expenditure is the misuse of the doctor's time by uninformed patients who have become irresponsible in respect of their health. They are incapable of knowing how to distinguish between what is serious and what is not (perhaps because the doctor has not shown enough confidence in them to tell them!), and they live in a country with social security, whose citizens have a 'right' to health as they have to owning the latest gadget ...

Look at the number of unnecessary home visits requested by patients who could perfectly well have gone to the doctor's consulting room! The doctor who is called out sees his waiting room full of patients who, after a few minutes, will choose not to wait any longer, for fear that their consultation will be rushed, and who will force the doctor to call on them at home without any real medical justification. Where will the vicious circle end?

As it is, many paediatricians no longer make home calls, and the majority of ENT specialists make the patients come to the surgery even in acute cases, for technical reasons.

'Misuse' of the doctor himself, reducing him to a prescriber of medicines, or of laboratory tests or X-rays is another cause of the squandering of resources. We need mention only the regulations which diminish a doctor to the rôle of 'distributer' of medicines which the patient himself has decided to have. Sometimes one has the unpleasant feeling that the prescriptions have become a sort of trading stamp, like those given away in service stations and supermarkets.

We do not want to dwell on the advertisements for certain medicines, which seems to attach more importance to the taste of antibiotic syrups than to what is in them, or which, for example, holds up as an example to grandchildren their dear little grandmother swallowing her tranquilisers! It does, however, seem important to remind ourselves that medicine represents only 18% of social-security expenses; so one cannot blame the whole problem on the consumption of medicines. It would rather seem that the hospitals are much more to blame, both in the cost of building and running them (since they are dependent on their daily fees) and in the way they are used, with whole lists of patients admitted unnecessarily or staying an unnecessarily long time.

Without failing to recognise the technical importance of hospitals—for diagnosis, for example, and especially for the treatment of certain well established conditions—and without denying the part they play in the field of surgery, it is necessary to adopt a new attitude towards them. Some general practitioners, who think it vitally important to 'dehospitalise' health, have already begun to take steps in this direction. With the help of a well chosen team, hospitalisation should be only one of the means of establishing a diagnois, making use of techniques unavailable in ordinary practice; but it would be a good thing if the doctor in charge of the case could take a part in deciding the therapy to be used. This is a problem which does not seem to be likely to be solved soon, even though certain services are making efforts in this direction.

These are not just the whinings of homoeopaths for whom 'there is no salvation outside their own church'. It is by analysing the positive and negative aspects of these problems that we underline the importance of our approach, for we know that our daily experience could be multiplied many times over and so make a real impact.

'Forewarned is Forearmed' is a Maxim Valid for Everyone
Because homoeopathy provides health education and because it

enables very many pathological conditions to be treated effectively right from the start with a few well tried remedies, it has given rise to a completely different approach to illness in current practice. This is in no way a question of encouraging people towards useless or dangerous self-medication, but of enabling them to be forewarned and so forearmed. One of us (like many of our fellow homoeopaths), in counselling his patients, has clearly seen the attitude of entire families being changed by first one person and then the whole group taking charge of their own health, thus leading to a considerable saving of money, especially where a large number of children with repeated attacks of nasopharyngitis had formerly placed a heavy strain on the family budget.

This attitude also makes it possible to know in good time when it is necessary to take more dramatic action, when the situation requires urgent technical medical help or the use of special methods of diagnosis. Thus, in a number of cases, unnecessary hospitalisation of the patient is avoided.

Furthermore, the practice of homoeopathy prevents accidents during treatment, which account for 5-20% of all hospital admissions (H. Pradal: *Les grands médicaments*, p. 42). Homoeopathic remedies are given in doses which are nontoxic (which is not to say that they are ineffective), and they stimulate the normal defence mechanisms of an organism affected by disease. They have no effect on a healthy organism, as has been shown by experiments on animals. Similarly, we avoid the risk of accidents caused by mixing and increasing the effect of medical substances (a current source of concern to the health authorities). It is a fact that too many sick people think that they can mix conventional medicines with impunity, and dose themselves without consulting a doctor.

Moreover, it should be possible to reserve heavy medication for cases where it is really necessary, and not to use a sledgehammer to crack a nut, as is done in 80% of the cases met within current practice. We are thinking, for example, of reactional depressive conditions, maintained and aggravated by an insane therapy which keeps the patient in his depression for years on end, when this could perfectly possibly have been avoided.

Time is another factor in favour of homoeopathy from the economic point of view. A patient treated for ten or fifteen years for a chronic condition is a long-term cost to society. Moreover, he has a tendency to develop intermittent acute attacks, from which he recovers more slowly if he is constantly under ill advised chemotherapy. If his condition is alleviated for six months or a year at a time, with, when the improvement has become established, the possibility of taking his remedies at greater intervals, he is no longer sick but well; and it is much cheaper both for him and for society if his equilibrium is maintained thereafter. The patient will be less subject to subsequent long, drawn-out acute conditions, since his resistance will no longer be dulled; and if, nevertheless, an operation should become necessary (even a serious one), it will, in the majority of cases, not lead to any ante- or post-operative problems. This is something we experience constantly with our patients. But, above all, let no one think that homoeopathy is a universal panacea, and that everything is always extraordinarily easy! However, the facts speak for themselves with apparent regularity among our respective patients. At any rate, let us not forget that we are speaking here of homoeopathy as a technique applying the law of similars and nothing else; this is to undertline the fact that it has nothing in common with its current image in official circles, for instance in the following report by Sournia:

Homoeopathic medicine has never been the subject of any statistical investigation and its effectiveness has never been proved. Yet many doctors make their living by it and, contrary to general opinion, its prescriptions are costly. Would a rational doctor prescribe many hundreds of thousand doses a year of suppositories made of brain-extract for children who do not get on well at school? (Freud and Bachelard would laugh their heads off!) Would a rational doctor prescribe calves' liver extract from male calves rather than female ones of the same age, the one being three times as expensive as the other? Would a rational doctor continue to write out 'special prescriptions' not in the pharmacopoeia, combining various products, each having its own danger, which he combines without thought, making the chemist crush up in his mortar pills which have been costly to produce, despite the fact that the pharmaceutical associations warn members of their professions against such practices? The Public Health authorities could, it is true, forbid them ...

Far be it from us to take issue with any of his remarks: he is right in everything he says. The only thing is—and this is important—the method he is criticising is *not homoeopathy at all* but a travesty of it used, for example, by those so-called homoeopaths who run slimming cures and are the delight of a certain ill informed section of the press. Against such 'homoeopaths' M. H. Nargeolet (head of the French central service for pharmaceuticals and medicines) speaks out in this recent warning (information meeting of the Committee of Pharmacists, Paris, April 1973):

I have no hesitation in stressing that your society is right, and I congratulate if for disassociating itself entirely from certain procedures. These consist, for many practitioners, in providing under the label of 'homoeopathy' medicines which have nothing at all to do with Hahnemann's doctrine. They are nothing more than allopathic preparations, formulated and prescribed without consideration of the risks run by patients and used in a kind of medicine which one can also describe as charlatanistic, since it covers practices highly criticisable from the point of view of medical ethics. I am speaking in particular about certain slimming or rejuvenating treatments, based on amphetamines or similar products, prescribed in dilutions which have nothing to do with homoeopathy.

I very much hope that your efforts, together with those of the association and of our own, will enable an end to be made to these abuses of the right of prescription and preparation.

It is not logical to criticise a method on the grounds of being something which it is not. 'A doctrine is not judged by its mistakes, but by its highlights,' Albert Camus said. It is, then, more a question of the information and the contacts you have.

Homoeopathy: 'yes'; Blunderbuss Therapy: 'no'

The price of a homoeopathic treatment is, without any doubt, one of the arguments in favour of the method, provided that it is not inflated by what one of our friends has called 'blunderbuss therapy'; that is by a mixture of remedies prescribed without rhyme or reason and almost, if not quite, as mad as those prescribed by some of our orthodox colleagues.

Indeed, the price of a three months' effective treatment of pure homoeopathy amounts to 18 francs (less than £2) per month for the patient and, what is more important, the improvement this brings him makes it possible to take the medicines at less frequent intervals and, thus, to reduce the lifetime of the chronic illness.

The moderate cost of the treatment depends, too, on the patient himself. We know that there are people who have a medical need to go on having treatment even when their equilibrium has been restored. In such cases it is possible for us deliberately to use a certain number of placebos in a homoeopathic form—a double paradox for those who think that all our remedies have a placebo effect!

IT IS COMPLICATED

Homoeopathy is supposed to be complicated. It is much more likely that it is the homoeopath himself who is complicating the practice of homoeopathy. Everyone has seen prescriptions containing fifteen or twenty different constituents to be taken every hour of the day. In some cases you would almost have to stay away from work in order to take them all. Unfortunately, such prescriptions are produced not just by certain homoeopaths: many other doctors are no less 'generous' with their exaggerated prescriptions.

It is their way of practising, a completely muddled method of choosing and prescribing medicines. More often than not these prescriptions are inexplicable, hence the confusion on the part of the patient and of the chemist, and sometimes even of the prescriber, if he is questioned about it.

It is possible with very few medicines—three to six at most, some reinforcing, others complementary—to give an effective homoeopathic treatment for any chronic disease. Certain of these medicines will be prescribed at certain stages of the disease according to the patient's basic constitution and his way of reacting. It is a question of technique and a method of prescribing medicines which is not as complicated as people imagine.

On the other hand, in a number of ordinary complaints you can employ homoeopathic medicines yourself. In this way you can carry out your own treatment intelligently, effectively, safely and with little trouble.

The only thing you must do at the beginning of a chronic illness is to take the pills regularly (but is it not just the same with orthodox medicines?). Thus for a cold you should take *Pyrogenium* every half-hour or every hour and *Belladonna* and *Ferrum phosphoricum* alternately every hour. As soon as the condition improves you can space out the remedies and then stop them altogether.

Thus it will be seen that the story that homoeopathic treatment is long, complicated and almost impossible to follow, with an impressive array of medicines which have to be changed all the time, is just pure invention.

CHAPTER V

Treat Yourself by Homoeopathy

Every acute or subacute illness starts off with signs which cause you a few hours' discomfort. At this stage—when your body is being attacked by a virus, a germ, some kind of food or a psychological upset—it responds by manifesting stress in an attempt to regain its equilibrium. Very often it manages this by itself and everything is put right again. Sometimes, though, the attack is too severe or is repeated too often and then the body needs help in order not to be overwhelmed. Homoeopathic remedies are there to help you to be 'forewarned and forearmed'. If the trouble is not cleared up quickly (we shall tell you in each case how long it should take), you should consult your doctor. Take good note of the general indications given for each situation. We do not want to give you primarily a chapter of 'recipes': we think you are capable of understanding the reasons why you should take such-and-such a remedy. We know that this attitude will be criticised, because we are giving you a number of 'keys'; but this risk must be taken. It is up to you to be independent and responsible for your own choice. For our part, we think it is only right and proper to treat you as a responsible, intelligent adult human being.

Let us recap briefly the essential points of the method:

Homoeopathy is a *therapeutic method* which uses on a sick person in *nontoxic doses* medical substances of mineral, vegetable or animal origin, which, if given in *toxic doses*, would produce in a healthy person a set of symptoms (or a syndrome) *similar* to the disease in question.

129

Homoeopathy

This method can be carried out very easily in practice by comparing two reactional syndromes:

- the reactional syndrome (of functional and/or lesional nature) observed in a healthy person, who has been given a strong or weak toxic dose;

- the reactional syndrome (of functional and or lesional nature) observed in a sick person, in response to somatic, infectious (by bacterium or virus), traumatic, alimentary, climatic or psychological attack.

Some Detail
Homoeopathic remedies are available in the following forms:
- tubes of pillules: 75 to the tube (quantity to be taken: 3 pillules at a time, to be repeated according to instructions)
- single-dose pills—200 pills to the gram (the whole dose to be taken at one time)
- Bottles of drops (10 to 15 drops to be taken at one time)

They are also available in all these forms:
- triturations
- suppositories
- liniments

The quantities are the same for babies, children, adults and old people: only the number of times the remedy is to be repeated or the dilution will vary according to circumstances.

In order to give you a practical understanding of the logic behind the choice of a particular homoeopathic remedy, we have invented the following scenario for your benefit. It will enable you to grasp serious ideas in what we hope is a light-hearted way.

SPORT AND HOMOEOPATHY

Introduction
Here is a little practical advice before you go on a winter-

sports holiday. We will tell you how to make up a little homoeopathic emergency kit, how to use it, and within what limits you should so so. This advice will enable you to become familiar with the remedies. For this purpose we will show you the correct 'responses' as we go along, so that you will know what to do and *what not to do*, and when it is advisable or even imperative to call in the doctor. We would like to remind you here that, if you want to choose a homoeopathic medicine in these everyday situations, you need to know the therapeutic effect of the remedy in question and various syndromes (groups of symptoms) which have been precisely described by homoeopaths as a result of their repeated experience. It is not a question of giving model prescriptions, but one of applying a method based on logical reasoning.

The Journey (nausea, vertigo, muscular pains)

'*The snow is falling* ... the train is moving on through the night ... Tomorrow you will be on the snow slopes ... '

(a) You find it difficult to sleep; you have always been bad at journeys (trains, 'planes, cars). You have a great deal of nausea, aggravated by the slightest movement. Your body breaks out in a cold sweat; fresh air makes you feel better. Your remedy is *Tabacum* 5c, 3 pills to be repeated every quarter of an hour, then less frequently as the condition improves.

Why?

Remember your first cigarette! Tobacco, through its active principle, nicotine, concentrates its action on the ganglions of the autonomic, sympathetic and parasympathetic systems, and produces these same symptoms.

You are nauseous, but *the dizziness is even worse*. You feel better when you are lying down and worse as soon as you leave the horizontal position. Your remedy is *Cocculus* 5c in the same dosage.

Why?

Cocculus Indicus, Indian Berry, contains picrotoxin, which produces the same syndrome by irritating the spinal cord.

These two short examples should enable you to grasp how to

131

reason by analogy. You are comparing *two reactional syndromes:* a reactional syndrome which can be produced in a healthy individual by nicotine or picrotoxin; and a similar reactional syndrome, travel sickness, observed in your case on a train journey.

The remedy will be either *Tabacum* or *Cocculus* according to the characteristics of your individual reaction. And yet, you have taken neither tobacco nor Indian berry! That is the homoeopathic way of reasoning it out.

You must consult a doctor if these troubles are frequent or very troublesome, since they may have their origin in an infection of the inner ear (or ENT) or malfunction of the liver.

(b) You have arrived; the bunks were rather hard and uncomfortable. Your back is sore; your muscles are painful and feel as if they had been bruised. Your remedy is *Arnica* 15c, 3 pillules

Why?

A strong dose of *Arnica montana* produces muscular pains and discoloration of the skin by acting on the blood vessels, giving rise to characteristic feelings of contusion and bruising. This syndrome is similar to the one observed as a result of injury (severe or slight, but repeated, as in the case of prolonged effort or a tiring journey). The remedy for these syndromes is therefore *Arnica*.

On the Snow Slopes (stage-fright, injuries, sprains)

(a) You are about to have your first skiing lesson. You are using the ski-lift. It's a long way off the ground! You are weak at the knees; you have pains in your stomach; you are trembling violently, which makes you clumsy. You've got stage-fright. Your remedy is *Gelsemium* 5c, 3 pillules as a preventative or during exercise.

Why?

A strong dose of yellow jasmine is a violent poison which acts on the cerebrospinal system and brings on paralysis of the motor nerves. It also produces violent trembling, aggravated by the slightest emotion. *Gelsemium*, then, is one of the remedies for stage-fright. It can also be useful in other circumstances (examinations, driving-tests, fear of journeys).

(b) *You are off*! (*Gelsemium* has done its work!) You keep having falls, not serious ones, but lots of them. On various parts of your body you have large and small bruises which feel painful. In addition, if you did not prepare for your holiday by doing exercises, your muscles will hurt as soon as you have to make an effort.

Your remedy is *Arnica* 15c, three times a day until you feel better.

(c) *'The sky's the limit!'* Your style is improving and consequently you are taking greater risks. You have a more serious fall.

Go to the doctor and have an X-ray if:

• after a strain or a sprain in any joint you feel a quick, violent pain accompanied by nausea and then, after a little lull, the pain comes back again.

• the pain is localised at one particular spot or if you have difficulty in moving the injured limb.

An X-ray is necessary in these two cases to make sure there is no serious sprain, no slight wrenching of the bone, no crack or fracture which might necessitate the limb being put in plaster. At the same time, a medicament can be of benefit right from the moment of injury—although, of course, this is additional to any necessary local treatment. The remedy is (again) *Arnica* 15c, 3 pillules every 10 minutes and then, after the pain has lessened, every half-hour, with a further 3 pills 3 times a day until you have completely recovered. In the case of a severe injury *Arnica* diminishes the effects of a possible shock to the cardiovascular system, and should be used in conjunction with orthodox treatment if necessary.

• in the case of cuts, *Calendula T.M.* as a disinfectant and while putting on dressings (25 drops in a glass of water), and *Pyrogenium* 3 times a day.

- in the case of a crack or fracture, it is worth using, in addition to *Arnica*, phosphate of lime: *Calcarea phosphorica* 15c, 3 pills 3 times a day; this encourages the formation of callus through its enhancement of the phosphorus-calcium metabolism.
- if a strain or sprain is still troublesome after you have taken *Arnica*, add poisonous sumac: *Rhus Toxicodendron* 7c, 3 pillules 3 times a day; this is a remedy for painful, inflamed joints where the condition is improved by movement and aggravated by damp; it acts on the tendons surrounding the joints.
- to make it less complicated, the remedies can be taken in groups 3 times a day, but leaving a quarter of an hour between each medicine: *Arnica-calcarea phosphorica* or *Arnica-Rhus Toxicodendron*.

Trip (burning, swelling, conjunctivitis, sunburn)

(a) You have avoided all these mishaps and are on the ski runs. The sun is shining, the snow is reflecting the light ... and you have forgotten your sunglasses. Your eyelids are swelling, pricking and burning; a little snow applied to them makes you feel better. Your remedy is *Apis* 15c, three pills every quarter of an hour, then, as soon as there is any improvement, progressively less frequently until the trouble has stopped.

Why?

Everyone has seen the effect of a bee-sting: the skin turns pale pink and it swells, pricks and burns, and the pain is ameliorated by cold. *Apis* is the remedy for inflammatory troubles dominated by swelling. In this instance it is the sun which has done the damage.

(b) You may have slightly different troubles: your eyelids are red, especially at the edges; you are blinking your eyes, the light hurts you; your conjunctivas are red, there is a little swelling: you have conjunctivits. Your remedy is *Belladonna* 5c.

Why?

A strong dose of belladonna produces acute or subacute

inflammatory congestion with spasms and hypersensitivity. A weaker dose of belladonna cures these complaints.

(c) You will understand at once that *Apis* will also be one of the essential remedies for the first stage of sunburn. At the second stage, when blisters appear (second-degree sunburn), the remedy is *Cantharis* 15c, three pillules every two hours, then progressively less frequently as the pain and the skin condition improve.

Why?

Through the medium of cantharidine, *Cantharis* has a blistering action on the digestive and especially the urinogenital mucous membranes, but also on the skin where, if it is taken, it produces injury similar to second-degree sunburn. *Cantharis* is the homoeopathic remedy.

Back to the Valley

At last you have left this hostile realm and are back again in the village. The day ends with some 'after-ski' activity, for which after your holiday you may perhaps need to take some doses of *Ignatia* 5c, the remedy for various spasmodic troubles which might arise after you've been crossed in love ...

It will be seen that among all these remedies the main ones and the most frequently indicated are *Apis* and *Arnica*, so take several tubes of pills of these, as well as *Arnica* ointment for local application. You will be able to use them on your friends who will be amazed to see that homoeopathic remedies can help them so quickly and so effectively, provided they are applicable in their particular case.

DIGESTIVE TROUBLES

With these, your approach should be the same as in all other cases: consult a doctor for *serious medical conditions;* and treat *simple troubles* yourself. We will describe the syndromes most frequently encountered in daily practice.

Indications
Consult a doctor in all digestive troubles if the pain is:

- regular; i.e., if it comes back every day at the same time with lulls lasting several days and then return of pain every day at the same time: it is possible that you have a duodenal or gastric ulcer;
- accompanied by haemorrhages, even if these are slight;
- accompanied by a feeling of blockage in the oesophagus or stomach;
- accompanied by vomiting which does not bring the patient any quick relief.

You should also go to the doctor at once for:

- any digestive syndrome with arthralgia (pain in the joints) and pruritis (itching) there is a possibility you have viral hepatitis;
- any syndrome with pain behind the breastbone and painful eructation (belching), especially in a young adult: this could be a heart attack.

Our Therapeutic Advice
You must definitely pay attention to your eating habits, the rhythm of your meals, the balance in their composition, the quality of the food, and faults in your diet which you did not know about (for example, intake of too much sugar leading to hypoglycaemia, the famous 'sinking feeling' at eleven o'clock. Very often a simple adjustment to the balance of your diet will allay your digestive troubles; but it is no good alleviating a trouble unless you act on the true cause.

People who take too many stimuli, who smoke or drink too much, will find their trouble recurring, even if it has been relieved by *Nux vomica* or by some allopathic remedy which acts in the same way.

What do your hear yourself saying?
'My digestion isn't working.'
'It won't go down.'

'I can't take anything.'
'I just don't know what to eat.'
'I never feel hungry when I'm annoyed.'

And so on. We can sum up all these situations in a few imaginary scenarios.

The Nux Vomica Syndrome

You have eaten too much too quickly and without chewing it. You take highly seasoned foods and stimulants. You are inclined to drink a little too much at meals. After the meal you have a feeling of heaviness at the pit of your stomach, you have acidity and nausea and above all you have a strong desire to go to sleep. Five or ten minutes' sleep will put everything right.

These troubles are often accompanied by a tongue coated at the back, a mistaken urge to defaecate, and a general state of irritability.

Strychnine, which is the main component of *Nux vomica*, is able to produce a similar syndrome in a healthy person. Here, since the bad eating habits are the cause, *Nux vomica* is the remedy.

Dosage: 5c, 3 pillules when the trouble occurs. To be repeated half-an-hour later if improvement does not come quickly; for a person disinclined to 'listen to reason', as a preventative, 3 pillules before meals will help digestion.

The Pulsatilla Syndrome

You take the pulsatilla anemone for indigestion caused by *fat, fatty foods and pastries*. People requiring *Pulsatilla* often suffer from circulatory troubles in their veins. It is the lessening of the flow of blood in their veins and the slowing down of digestion in the mucous lining of the stomach which cause the dyspepsia.

Dosage: 5c, 3 pillules to be taken when the trouble starts. To be repeated half-an-hour later, if necessary.

The Antimonium Crudum Syndrome

This corresponds to the person who eats too much. His tongue is white, and he is prone to diarrhoea. He frequently has

137

eczema or skin troubles. Remember, this is the *glutton* type.

Dosage: 5c, 3 pillules when the trouble starts. Repeat as necessary.

The Robinia Syndrome

This is very simple, but the remedy acts very quickly on people with 'acidity' at the pit of the stomach, often accompanied by aching at the front of the head.

The Chelidonium Syndrome

In this case it is the gall bladder which is not functioning properly. The sign of this is a pain on the right side, quite close to the pit of the stomach, but the fact that it comes from the gall bladder is shown by the way the pain stretches right up to the point of the right shoulder blade.

There is often headache just above the eye, the tongue is coated and damp, there is nausea and the stools are slightly discoloured.

Dosage: 5c, 3 pillules at the onset of pain. Repeat as required.

These few simple suggestions will help you to cope with everyday troubles; they will aslo assist you not to overlook more serious illness if you always *do the right thing when the trouble starts.*

You may, of course, have an attack of itching or yawning due to nerves, calling for a dose of *Ignatia,* but at the same time you may be suffering from viral hepatitis, requiring you to call in the doctor. In this way you will have helped him in his difficult task!

INTESTINAL TROUBLES

You have intestinal trouble. What *must* you do? What *can* you do? We shall confine ourselves to outlining situations which you may experience daily without entering into learned definitions of exact medical diagnoses which might serve only to confuse you. The best help we can give you is to show you not only your *limits* but also your *possibilities.*

Indications

You must consult your doctor in the following cases:

- Diarrhoea which does not improve in 24 or 48 hours although you are taking the prescribed remedies. If there is no positive reaction, then the cause is more by rooted or the remedies are insufficient.

  Special case: never delay in the case of a baby or a very young child, since dehydration sets in rapidly at this age. It is necessary to rehydrate the child with intravenous infusion.

  However, *Veratrum album* can help while waiting for the doctor to come or for the patient to be taken to hospital. In some cases, of course, there is no doctor or hospital near at hand (in countries with poor medical facilities, or where distances are great).

- Diarrhoea with nausea and vomiting, shivering, temperature 38-39°C (100-102°F). It may be an acute attack of angiocholitis (inflammation of the bile ducts due to a stone), serious microbial infection of the intestine or sometimes appendicitis (although this usually gives temporary constipation).

- Chronic diarrhoea, which necessitates the exact cause being found. The doctor will make a general check-up, but will also need to examine your stools and X-rays of your intestines, and will go on to make a local examination in order to look for an infection, a disease caused by parasites, a tumour (polyp), and endocrine troubles: diarrhoea is sometimes a sign of the malfunction of the thyroid gland.

- Beware of false diarrhoea brought on by laxatives, which make you lose a large amount of potassium in the stools and bring on muscular cramp. This condition requires a serious medical examination.

- Constipation which has set in recently, especially if it alternates with periods of diarrhoea.

What You Can Do

Fortunately, the situation is usually less 'dramatic'. You can use several remedies, thus being forewarned and forearmed, and this will often be sufficient in itself. We will, therefore, describe to you simply a few syndromes (collections of symptoms) which will enable you to choose the right remedy.

Veratrum Album Syndrome

Diarrhoea, vomiting, cold sweat on the forehead (a very characteristic sign), sometimes dizziness during or after defaecation. Very frequently seen after food-poisoning by oysters or mussels, but also occurring in other infections.

Remember Hippocrates, and apply the law that 'like is cured by like', and treat choleric syndromes with this remedy. Dosage: 5c, 3 pillules after each abnormal defaecation until cured.

Podophyllum Syndrome

Podophyllin is a very drastic substance which produces violent diarrhoea, aggravated by the slightest intake of liquid or solid food, and often accompanied by gurgling and pain in the hollow of the right hip bone. It is often used in teething (like *Chamomilla*, but without irritability).

Dosage: 15c (this dilution seems to be more effective), 3 pillules after each abnormal defaecation.

Arsenicum Album Syndrome

Diarrhoea, vomiting, thirst for cold water which is vomited as soon as it is warmed up in the stomach (as with *Phosphorus*). Rapid alteration of the general condition. Remedy for serious food-poisoning by bad food. Consult your doctor at once if there is no improvement. Sometimes nervous agitation.

Dosage: 5c, 3 pillules after each abnormal defaecation.

China Syndrome
A large quantity of diarrhoea, painless, with much wind and distention. Sometimes a little expistaxis (nose-bleeding).
Dosage: 5c, 3 pillules after each abnormal stool.

Gelsemium Syndrome
Diarrhoea with shivering and muscular pain. Trembling; absence of thirst in spite of fever. This is a viral syndrome.
Dosage: 15c, 3 pillules every hour, then less frequently after general improvement.
Nervous diarrhoea before exams, due to 'stage-fright'.
Dosage: 9c, one dose the night before, and 5c, 3 pillules at each abnormal defaecation.

Paratyphoidinum B15c
A biotherapy to be taken systematically in conjunction with each of these remedies, especially in the case of food-poisoning by oysters or mussels.
Dosage: 1 dose every 8 hours (a course of 3 doses).

Constipation Is a Special Problem
It is an illness which should be treated seriously. It is necessary to call in the doctor. A homoeopathic remedy by itself is not sufficient to cure this problem: it is necessary to consider the patient's whole constitution.

EAR, NOSE AND THROAT TROUBLES

You must bear in mind *two essential points*:
- Early treatment with a few simple, easily prescribed remedies can avoid complications, possibly serious ones, although the situation may have appeared perfectly commonplace at the beginning.
- It is necessary and possible to adjust a constitution predisposed to these troubles by means of homoeopathic therapy. Why and how does a doctor act in such a case? We will explain this to you.

141

What Ought You To Know About Nose and Throat Troubles in Children?

These are the expression of an inflammatory condition of the upper respiratory apparatus (nose, pharynx) and are due to viruses or germs. They often occur at the same time as changes in the weather.

The mucous membranes of the respiratory tract are attacked and react in several successive stages: congestion, swelling, inflammation, reactive secretion which can lead to further infection with lesions of the tissues (erosion or ulceration of the mucous membrane and bleeding).

Sometimes these troubles clear up of their own accord, but the risk is that they may lead to complications involving the nearby organs (ears, larynx, tonsils, bronchi). They may also be the beginning, the initial stage of one of the diseases of childhood.

The Indications for General Medical Care

Consult the doctor or the ENT specialist in the following cases:

- otalgia (earache), where the child is exhausted between each paroxysm of pain, since there is the possibility of deep suppuration requiring an operation on the eardrum;
- sudden discharge from the ear;
- the onset of a feeling of dizziness or of a cough with pain in the chest;
- increase in temperature, even though the correct remedies appear to have been used.
- accompanying ganglions in the neck or at the back of the head, (possibility of rubella—german measles—or glandular fever);
- and, above all, when there is no obvious improvement within forty-eight hours of taking the remedies.

This apparently harmless trouble if taken lightly at the beginning may lead to serious complications. It is important to have some simple indications of what to do *during the first few hours*. It is at this stage that *true prevention* can take place.

Be Forewarned and Forearmed

(a) *What you can do at a very early stage*

- *Onset*

  Dry cold. Swiftness of onset. Sneezing. sometimes raised temperature without sweating. The child is congested, sometimes restless and upset. *Aconite* 5c.

  Dry cold. Wind. Feeling of obstruction in the nose. Shivering at the slightest movement and on taking off clothes. Sometimes irritability. *Nux vomica* 5c.

  Damp cold. Catches cold after having been soaked by rain—this often happens to children in foggy weather. Sometimes ganglions (swellings) in the neck or at back of the head. *Dulcamara* 5c.

- *The troubles should diminish within a few hours*

  If not, the next stage is a discharge. In this case the remedy must be changed, according to the following scheme:

  THE DISCHARGE IS IRRITATING

  Much sneezing. The eyes are tearful, but do not irritate: *Allium cepa* 5c.

  Much irritation with a burning sensation. Excoriations, little sores in the nostrils. Local and general improvement through warmth. *Arsenicum album* 5c.

  Greenish-yellow discharge; evil-smelling. Tongue coated. Salivation. Foul breath. Sometimes shivering and night sweats. *Mercurius solubilis* 5c.

  THE DISCHARGE IS NOT IRRITATING

  Eyes irritated. This picture corresponds to the initial stage of german measles. *Euphrasia* 5c.

  Plentiful discharge, yellow, free-flowing; very much aggravated by hot rooms, much improved by fresh air. The more clothes you put on the children, the more they 'excrete'. You must make them go out into the fresh air. *Pulsatilla* 5c.

  Yellow discharge, but thick, will not flow easily. Improvement in heat. *Hydrastis* 5c.

- The throat becomes painful when swallowing. *Belladonna* 5c. *Mercurius solubilis* 5c. *Pyrogenium* 7c.

- A cough appears
  Very dry, aggravated by a warm room. *Ferrum phosphoricum*
  5c. *Bryonia* 5c. (3 pillules alternately every two hours.)
  Very loose, with nausea. *Ferrum phosphoricum* 5c. *Ipeca* 5c.
  (Alternately every 2 hours.)

- The nose bleeds. *China* 5c. *Millefolium* 5c. (Alternately
  every 10 minutes.)

- The ear is painful. *Belladonna* 5c. *Ferrum phosphoricum* 5c
  every 2 hours. *Pyrogenium* 7c 3 times a day. *Capsicum* 7c
  once in the afternoon.

- In the special case of hayfever it is *always necessary* to
  consult a doctor. You may be helped by alternating two
  remedies which are often indicated: *Apis* 15c and *Pulmonary
  histamine* 15c, 3 pillules alternately every half hour, then less
  frequently when there is improvement.
  You should know that an acute attack is often difficult to
  calm down with homoeopathic remedies. In the circumstances an orthodox therapy may be more suitable and may
  act more quickly. On the other hand, a large part is played
  by the patient's constitution, so you should consult a
  homoeopath.

(b) Some general advice
In every case, in order to prevent possible infectious complications, you can systematically give in addition: *Pyrogenium* 7c, 3
pillules 3 times a day. The action of this remedy is one of non-
specific stimulation in the case of infectious troubles.

- Take the remedy indicated in the dilution 5c, 3 pillules
  every half hour or every hour according to the severity of the
  case. On improvement, extend the interval to one hour, then
  two hours. Leave off when the trouble has stopped for at
  least four hours.

- If the initial picture is not clear, alternate between *Belladonna* 5c and *Ferrum phosphoricum* 5c (3 pillules alternately every hour). This is frequently effective, since these remedies correspond to the symptoms at the beginning of every inflammatory condition: congestion, swelling, spasm, inflammation, and a slight tendency towards bleeding. In addition they make it possible for you to protect the ears, *Ferrum phosphoricum*, in particular, having the ability to produce a specific response from these organs.

(c) Why should attention be given to constitution?
Everyone knows how inevitably these troubles become chronic, how they keep recurring constantly, so that antibiotics and perhaps even corticosteroids have to be used, followed by surgical operations (to remove tonsils or adenoids). Yet is is possible to avoid these constant relapses by homoeopathic treatment of the constitution. A general, but simple, explanation is necessary here.

The body sustains attacks (viruses and germs are directly responsible for nose and throat troubles), and it reacts to these by stress—a non-specific defensive reaction—which enables it to adapt, to find a new system of balance so that it is able to defend itself. If this stress is too frequently required or is too intense, the organism no longer has the 'capacity to compensate'. It is then that the disease will appear, apparently as a result of a very slight cause—a change in the weather, bad diet, unfavourable psychological conditions.

You will understand, then, that it is possible to act on the external factors (germs, with doses varied according to the circumstances) and on the internal factors (stimulation of the natural defences of a constitution, which is predisposed towards the disease and no longer has the capacity to undertake its own defence).

This constitution, this predisposition towards such and such a disease, is made up of several elements. The individual is sensitive both biologically and by character, and this sensitivity is modified to a greater or lesser extent by heredity and by his own previous history. It is now known that it is possible to

145

group certain individuals according to such predispositions.

The study of tissue groups by the H.L.A. system (the work of Professor Dausset) shows there is a real *biochemical basis* for this type of constitution. This is expressed clinically as the individual reaction of the patient, which corresponds to the say the subject reacts to an attack.

It is essential to understand that the prescription of a homoeopathic remedy is made in answer to a *syndrome* of well coordinated reactions; it is a collection of symptoms, not just one single symptom, which characterises the way a disease manifests itself in a sick person.

If we seem to dwell on these definitions, it is because the doctor's diagnosis and therapy are based on these elements so that he can find the practical homoeopathic remedy for this constitution.

An example which is often encountered in practice is *silicea.* The child who responds to silicea has the following characteristics.

Build: Appearance close to the classic description of rickets. Thin with well developed frontal lobes.

Character: Easily tired, timid, irritable, needs to be stimulated. He often has problems in his relationship with his mother, feeling that she has abandoned him. You all know children like that, who were put into hospital at a very young age or had one nurse after another, and who have repeated nose and throat problems. This syndrome, a classic case, has even been described by paediatricians under the name 'child-as-left-luggage syndrome'.

History: Frequent chronic suppuration and growing troubles, of post-vaccinatory reactions. These are children in whom smallpox vaccination and the B.C.G. 'do not take'.

From the immunisation point of view they have a deficiency of immunoglobulin: 1gA

Their personal reaction: chilly, made worse by the cold. They perspire from the nape of the neck and the feet. Wounds heal with difficulty.

146

This is just a quick survey of one syndrome to let you know how a doctor's mind has been working when he finally decides to prescribe *Silicea*.

A Very Important Idea: Time

In the case cited above, high dilutions of 15c and 30c are necessary in order to produce a deep, gentle and lasting effect. Of course, a constitution does not let itself get out of order in a week and so it takes time to put it back into order again; but, with a simple technique, the results should be quite quick. It usually takes two months for the attacks to cease or become less acute.

After that it will be enough to maintain the child's dynamic balance by continuing to give it a constitutional remedy according to the medical situation.

This idea of *time* is of prime importance in every therapy.
Homoeopathy acts quicky when it is properly applied and the right dilutions are used. It is all a question of technique in treatment. It is for this reason that we think you should know about all these ideas.

BEHAVIOURAL PROBLEMS IN A CHILD

In the particular case of behavioural problems in a child, this is what we would advise you to do:

(a) General medical indications

- Consult a doctor when the troubles have appeared recently, with changes in the child's general condition (appetite, thirst, sweat, loss of weight, digestive troubles), if these are serious or become progressively worse.
- Have a complete medical examination carried out if the following troubles appear: repeated headaches, especially if they are accompanied by nausea; troubles with eyesight; very marked aggressiveness of recent origin and without apparent cause.
- Take medical advice of a psychological nature in the case of troubles which you know may perhaps be connected

situation of conflict in the family. Although there is often a lot of prejudice against psychologists, a competent one can be very valuable in revealing and resolving certain cases of conflict in which the child is involved.

(b) Our homoeopathic advice

You cannot and should not make a diagnosis of the disease or of the syndrome. We will, therefore, describe to you very systematically some everyday situations which you may well encounter.

We can, in general terms, define two main groups:—

- children who are calm but timid or inhibited,
- children who are restless or hyperactive.

Here we can only indicate temporary remedies which you can give without fear of upsetting the constitutional treatment prescribed by your local homoeopathic doctor. Proper treatment of such children should be concerned with the whole unbalanced psychosomatic state.

Calm Timid Children

- *Ambra grisea*: Often indicated for the *Pulsatilla* or *Silicea* type. Hypersensitive, blushing readily at the slightest emotion; dislikes strange faces and is afraid when the focus of attention is on him. Prefers to play alone or with a few friends, often of similar disposition. In general, sensitive to smells, as *Ignatia*.

  Dosage: 15c; 3 granules 3 times a day when the condition is bad.

- *Gelsemium*: Well known: the 'stagefright' type. Emotionally caused diarrhoea before going to school, with abdominal spasms, especially if there is an exam in the offing. The sort of pupil who hands in a blank piece of paper, in contrast to the *Argentum nitricum* type who, in his hurry, fails to read the question properly before answering.

  This is often a remedy for a child of the *Sepia* or *Pulsatilla* type.

Dosage: 7c; 3 granules when the symptoms occur. Repeat at your discretion according to improvement of the symptoms.

- *Ignatia*: More lively, less inhibited than the *Gelsemium* type. This child is more susceptible to emotions, to irritation and to extroverted displays of affection. The reactions are more spectacular, but more superficial—more ' theatrical'.
  The child will complain of various and changing aches and pains, often of an impossible nature: the essential characteristic is that they all disappear as soon as someone takes an interest or the atmosphere is congenial to him.

Dosage: 7c; 3 granules when the pains arise.

Restless Hyperactive Children
In practice, these children are more frequently encountered. It is quite possible, without turning them into vegetables, to help them live in harmony with their temperaments using the following remedies:

- *Chamomilla*: Quick-tempered and irritable, this type can be awkward and has a low irritation threshold, both with others and with themselves. Their actions are directed by mood; they throw their things around, eventually destroying them, and bang the doors.
  They are very sensitive to wind and bad-weather, are more irritable when the atmospheric pressure is low. However, their outbursts of anger are superficial and are really a way of expressing a certain basic anxiety and difficulty in communicating with those around them. This behaviour is found in the basic remedies most often indicated for such children: *Chamomilla*, *Lycopodium* and *Natrum muriaticum*, among others.

Dosage: 15c, 3 granules when the trouble occurs.

- *Nux vomica*: The children concerned are much more violent in their outbursts. The anger is accompanied by swearing and a tendency to hit out at and attack people around them.

149

Such children are, very often victims of digestive problems linked to improper diet. In short, it is the attribute of violence which causes us to turn to *Nux vomica*. Note that such children should always see a child psychologist.

Dosage: 7c; 3 granules at the time of the outburst.

- *Tarentula hispana*: Here we have a restless, agitated child, forever on the move. The basic way of inducing calm is through music—a medium easy to introduce in today's pop culture. Note that in the *Chamomilla* type it is movement which improves the mental state—walking, swaying regularly, travelling on vehicles etc.

Dosage: 15c; 3 granules 3 times a day.

A Special Case: 'Night Terrors'
At certain ages nightmares are normal phenomena. Only if they become too sleep-disturbing should you use the following treatments.
- *Belladonna*: The child screams and his face is covered in sweat. He has trouble waking up, and thinks that he sees animals, ghosts and terrifying figures.

Dosage: 15c; 3 granules at bedtime and at the time of distress. Note that this child often needs *Calcarea carbonica* as a constitutional remedy. Though impressionable, he greatly likes stories or entertainments which frighten him.

- *Stramonium*: A need for the child to have the light on at night indicates this remedy. In daytime such children are often aggressive, with a tendency to scratch or bite their friends.

Dosage: 15c; 3 granules at bedtime and when required.

- *Kali bromatum*: This child is full of movement throughout the day; the hands, in particular, are never still. He has to touch everything, to move things. He sleepwalks. Also he often has acne.

Dosage: 15c; 3 granules, 3 times a day.

These brief notes should give you everyday help. Do not forget to consider treatment if the symptoms do not clear up quickly or if the problems recur after temporary improvement.

DENTAL PROBLEMS IN CHILDREN

Children's dental problems occur on two levels:

- *Those related to the constitution in which they occur*: it is the job of the doctor to prescribe the indicated remedies. However, it is useful for *you* to know the underlying reasons for his prescription, so that you don't feel left in the dark.
- *Those related simply to dentition*: a number of simple remedies can be used.

The Constitution
Let us take two examples:

A thickset, square-featured baby-competition-winning type who is backward in teething. The doctor diagnoses swollen tonsils and adenoids, a tendency to recurring nasal catarrh, weeping eczema and sore bottom. The child has a big appetite and a predilection for sugar and indigestible foods. While sleeping he sweats from the scalp and he tends to have worms. The constitutional remedy, indicated by the clinical picture, is *Calcarea carbonica*.

In our second example the child's dental development is slow; but in this case it forms part of a more marked picture of underdevelopment. The morphological type recalls the classic rickets type. He is a sickly, crybaby, and sweats a lot from the nape of the neck and the feet even before weaning. This skinny child has little appetite and cannot tolerate milk. He is subject to running sores and reacts badly to vaccinations and to chemotherapy, even when this is appropriate. The constitutional remedy is *Silicea*.

151

Homoeopathy

The choice of prescription and of dilution is in the doctor's province; in general he will use 15c or 30c. The clinical picture is complete: a syndrome of dental retardation with precise antecedents, morphological type and exact characteristics. The parallel between the symptom picture observed and the *materia medica* is close.

Teething Troubles

In general terms, all dental growth may be accompanied by an inflammatory reaction with repercussions for the child's body as a whole. Once again, you'll find that familiar remedies are indicated: *Belladonna, Ferrum Phosphoricum* and *Aconite*. If the child is extremely irritable, but can be calmed by being carried or rocked, you will again find that *Chamomilla* is indicated. This remedy is even more strongly indicated if there is accompanying earache.

These remedies are given in a dilution of 5c and a dose of 3 granules, frequently repeated, according to results and the time taken for improvement to occur. Lt us remind you once again that the doctor's advice should be sought if the trouble persists, even if the remedy being given seems entirely appropriate.

Digestive problems and diarrhoea are frequent accompaniments to teething. There are two essential remedies to know:

- *Podophyllum*: The child salivates far too much and the least intake of food—or, more especially, liquid (orange juice, for example)—causes the stools to be released uncontrollably.

  Dosage: 15c; 3 granules for each abnormal stool, as a first-aid measure while awaiting the doctor's advice.

Always be aware of the seriousness of diarrhoea in weaning infants. Follow to the letter the doctor's advice concerning digestive problems.

- *Chamomilla*: Well known to you! The stools look like scrambled eggs—this appearance is very characteristic. Once again, irritability is calmed by movement.

Dosage: 9c or 15c according to the intensity of the nervous condition; 3 granules repeated frequently according to results.

Quite deliberately, we do not suggest any other remedies. The ones we have mentioned have stood the test of time: their clinical effectiveness has been demonstrated again and again. You can use them as a first measure without further consideration. Building on this solid foundation, you should be perfectly able to complete your knowledge.

PROBLEMS IN SLEEPING

Remember these three essential points:

- insomnia is a symptom whose cause must be located;
- our advice is based on a few very simple ideas;
- if improvement does not occur quickly (in a fortnight) go to your doctor so that he can put the 'biological clock' right.

General Medical Considerations

Go straight to the doctor in the following cases:

- *Insomnia with recent weight loss.* Here are the possible beginnings of a serious state of depression or of endocrinal illness (diabetes, for example).

- *Insomnia with profuse sweating.* This might indicate serious microbial infection—for example, tuberculosis or brucellosis if there are accompanying muscular pains.

- *Insomnia with cramp* at night in the calves: here there is the chance of potassium—related metabolic problems.

- *Insomnia necessitating the taking of medicinal substances in ever-increasing doses to ever-decreasing effect.* Another therapeutic answer must be found.

- *Recent excessive need for sleep*, particularly if there are associated visual problems. Look for a brain-related cause, and have a complete opthalmological examination.

- *Sleepwalking*. This condition often necessitates a neurological examination (electroencephalogram).

Our Advice is Twofold

Advice About Right Living

This might appear obvious, but it is worth reminding a 'new' insomniac about it. The rhythm of his or her life is often the cause, and there are imbalances in diet to be corrected.

Refer to the advice for fatigue—the two syndromes are often the same.

There are certain remedies which you can use according to circumstances

In all cases: *Passiflora* 1DH, 10 drops in a little water on retiring; or *Valeriana* 1DH, same dosage. These remedies help you get to sleep, and the dose can be repeated if you wake in the night without affecting the way you wake up.

Insomnia accompanied by mental hyperactivity: You have trouble in getting to sleep.

(a) Nux vomica syndrome: after abuse of stimulants (food, coffee, alcohol, tobacco) in a hyperactive person. Light sleep. Wakes up frequently and deep sleep comes 10 minutes before it is time to get up: 3 granules of 5c at dinner.

(b) Ignatia syndrome: as a result of distress, emotion and worry, in a person hypersensitive to all three. 3 granules of 5c at dinner.

(c) Chamomilla syndrome: irritable through lack of sleep, no tolerance to petty annoyances, a need to move and a feeling better for movement. This sort of insomniac can sleep in a train or a car; in the same category are children who go to sleep quickly on being rocked. 3 granules of 9c on retiring and on waking up during the night.

Insomnia with physical distress:

(a) Wakes between midnight and 2am feeling anxious, afraid of dying, desire to drink cold water, physical restlessness. *Arsenicum album* 9c, 3 granules at bedtime.

(b) Wakes about 3am with difficulty in breathing, as if suffering from asthma. Anxious, with cold sweats. Needs to sit down and remain still. *Kali carbonicum* 9c, 3 granules on retiring.

(c) Wakes about 4am with abdominal pains relieved by breaking wind. *Lycopodium* 5c, 3 granules on retiring and then on waking at the time of distress.

An excessive need for sleep, with much digestive trouble (swallowing air, swelling up). *Nux moschata* 9c, 3 granules before the two main meals.

For sleepwalking only: one remedy has often been found very useful: *Kali bromatum* 15c, 3 granules on retiring. Note, though, that this must be complemented by constitutional treatment.

Insomnia with nightmares which awaken the subject.

(a) Fear of the dark, and the need for light nearby. *Stramonium* 15c, 3 granules on retiring.

(b) The need for complete darkness. *Hyoscymus* 15c, 3 granules on retiring.

(c) Wakening with sweat around the head; often difficulty in waking up. *Belladonna* 15c, 3 granules on retiring.

Basic treatment is essential for long-lasting action when dealing with sleeping problems; such problems are often the first alarm bell indicating an imbalance in the body.

TIREDNESS

General Medical Considerations

First of all one should distinguish chronic fatigue from passing or occasional phases of tiredness. In the first case, a doctor's advice and diagnosis should always be sought, for fatigue can be a sign of serious illness; in the second, you can give help and advice.

If the state of tiredness persists for weeks then it is time to consult a doctor, particularly if it is accompanied by loss of weight, great thirst, pangs of hunger, sweating during the night, insomnia, temperature changes, swelling of the joints (even if only slight), a recent cough or chronic digestive problems.

The doctor will call for blood tests and X-rays to help detect

- anaemia (the cause must be found)
- a deep seated infection (a urinary infection, for example)
- an infectious disease (tuberculosis, brucellosis)
- diabetes or a condition of the endocrine glands (the adrenal glands, for example)
- a parasite
- the beginnings of depression.

Our Advice is Twofold

Advice About Right Living

A temporary state of tiredness is often related to bad diet or a bad physical or even psychological regime. Some alterations to your diet will help, for example, to avoid 'hypoglycemic phases'—that famous sinking feeling.

It is important to have breakfast and during the day, balanced meals with sufficient intake of calcium and magnesium: many cases of tiredness are linked solely to metabolic problems concerned with magnesium and phospho-calcium.

156

Remedies for Temporary Tiredness

After physical exertion:

(a) Effort involving muscles (sport, long walks, repeated traumatism, even minimal—journeys, for example): You feel bruised, as if you have been hit. Physical contact is painful, and insomnia frequent. *Arnica* 15c, 3 granules 3 times a day.

If pain is chiefly in the joints, but without swelling, and is the worse for rest, the better for movement: *Rhus toxicodendron* 9c, 3 granules 3 times a day.

(b) Illnesses with loss of organic liquid (bleeding, diarrhoea, vomiting). *China* 5c, 3 granules 3 times a day.

(c) When growing, or when bone is knitting after a fracture: *Calcarea phosphorica* 15c, 3 granules 3 times a day.

After Psychological Exertion

(a) Emotion, repeated worry, grief: Ambra grisea 15c, 3 granules 3 times a day (hypersensitivity and exacerbated timidity in these states). *Ignatia* 7c, 3 granules 3 times a day (frequent spasms of the 'lump in the throat' type, assorted and paradoxical problems).

(b) Intellectual overexertion: You are easily tired and irritable, lymphatic, and sweating readily from head to feet with the onset of tiredness. *Kali phosphoricum* 5c, 3 granules 3 times a day (loss of memory, and white phosphate deposits in the urine. *Anacardium* 9c, 3 granules 3 times a day (character problems: anger, indecision and loss of memory). *Silicea* 9c, 3 granules 3 times a day.

A remedy to use if the tiredness follows a period of physical and psychological overload in a hyperactive subject who abuses stimulants to keep up to the mark and then tries to recover with a ten-minute snatch of sleep: *Nux Vomica* 5c, 3 granules 3 times a day.

Homoeopathy

In All Cases of Tiredness, or if There is no Particular Indication

Coca 36DH; 10 drops in a little water on rising and at midday is an excellent remedy.

Overall

- chronic fatigue requires medical diagnosis.
- the way you eat is important

PAINS

Rheumatic Pains

The doctor should be consulted every time the pain with accompanying fever or cough, wakes you up at night.

Pains in the joints

Worse on rising, better for movement: *Rhus toxicodendron* 7c. Better for rest: *Bryonia* 7c. Worse in the damp: *Dulcamara* 7c, 3 times a day.

Muscular pains

In the back (after ironing, typing): *Cimicifuga* 7c, 3 times a day. Crick in the neck: *Lachnantes* 3c, 5 drops 3 times a day.

Osteoarthritis

At time of crisis basic treatment may be supplemented with:

Cervical arthritis: *Ferrum phosphoricum* 5c. Dorsal arthritis: *Ferrum phosphoricum* 5c: *Cimicifuga* 5c. Lumbar arthritis: *Ferrum phosphoricum 5c, Kali carbonicum* 5c.

Conclusion

Within the limits of what we have described, you can treat yourself with homoeopathic remedies for a number of everyday problems, as those who already do so will know. Those who do not now have the opportunity to try, without the risk of poisoning themselves to treat their everyday ills intelligently. Such ills can become much more serious if neglected and left to their natural development; on the other hand they can be 'overtreated' grossly in a way quite unnecessary at this stage. In our opinion, based on many years' trial and error in daily practice, the experience is well worth a try ...

YOUR OWN SMALL HOMOEOPATHIC PHARMACY

This list has been drawn up according to the advice we gave in the last chapter. On your own you must only use containers of granules: the other ways of taking remedies are best dealt with by your doctor. It is easy to carry with you the remedies you mentioned in the list.

It is right that you should know what you are using as medicines. The Latin name, which is the international homoeopathic name, is followed by the common name and the kingdom to which the substance belong: mineral (M), vegetable (V) or animal (A). We then list the part of the plant or animal used to make the remedy, and where relevant, its geographical provenance. The mineral substances are those commonly found in nature.

ACONITE 5c: Aconite (V)
　This plant is picked in August, towards the end of its
　flowering season, in the Vosges mountains in France, in
　Germany and in Switzerland.
ALLIUM Cepa 5c: Onion. (V)
　The fresh bulb of the onion.
AMBRA GRISEA 15c: Ambergris (A)
　Intestinal concretions from sperm-whales.
ANACARDIUM 15c: Ambergis (A)
　Dried fruit of a tree from the mountains of India.
ANTIMONIUM CRUDUM 5c: Sulphur of antimony (M)
APIS MELLIFICA 15c: (A)

159

The whole bee is put in alcohol, crushed and then macerated.

ARNICA MONTANA 15c: Wild arnica (V)

The whole plant is gathered when flowering (July and August) in the mountains of the Auvergne, the Vosges and Switzerland.

ARSENIGUM ALBUM 7c: Arsenious oxide (M)

BELLADONA 5c-15c: Deadly nightshade (v)

The whole plant is picked during the flowering season in June. It is found throughout Europe: in shady ditches, along hedgerows and in coppiced woods.

BRYONIA 5c: Briony (v)

A plant of the hedgerows. The berries are red or black.

CAESIUM 5c: Rare metal (M)

CALCAREA PHOSPHORICA 15c: Calcium phosphate (M)

CALENDULA: Marigold (v)

A common field plant in Europe.

CANTHARIS 15c: Coleoptea (beetles) (A)

The whole beetle is pulverised. The insect lives in the South of France, Spain and Italy on ash, honeysuckle, privet and lilac.

CHAMOMILLA 15c: Feverfew (v)

The whole plant; it grows in dry, sandy locations.

CHELIDONIUM 5c: Celandine (v)

The whole plant, which is found along hedgerows, old walls and in uncultivated sites throughout Europe.

CHINA 5c: Red quinquina (v)

The dried bark of a tree discovered in Peru in 1638.

CIMICIFUGA 7c

A perennial plant found in woods; has either follicles or berries. Common throughout Europe.

COCCULUS 5c: Indian Berry (v)

Dried fruit of a shrub found in India, Sri Lanka and Malaysia.

DULCAMARA 5c: Woody nightshade (v)

Leaves and stems picked before flowering. The plant is found in damp ditches, hedges and along river banks.

EUPHRASIA 5c: Eye-bright (v)

The whole, fresh plant, including root.

FERRUM PHOSPHORICUM 5c: Iron phosphate (M)
GELSEMIUM 7c: Trumpet creeper (V)
   Fresh root of a shrub from Virginia
HYDRASTIS 5c: Golden seal (V)
   Fresh root of a plant from Canada.
HYOSCYAMUS 15c: Henbane (V)
   The whole plant is picked in July. Found amongst rubble
   and on road verges.
IGNATIA 5c
   Seeds of a climbing plant from the Philippines.
IPECA 5c: Ipecacuanha (V)
   A plant of Indian origin
KALI BROMATUM 15c: Potassium bromide (M)
KALI CARBONICUM 9c: Potassium carbonate (M)
KALI PHOSPHORICUM 5c: Potassium phosphate (M)
LYCOPODIUM 5c: Club moss (V)
   The pollen of the moss, which grows especially in
   Germany and Switzerland, in woods and shaded sites.
MERCURIUS SOLUBILS 5c: Purified mercury (M)
   The seed of a shrub from India and Sri Lanka.
NUX MOSCHATA : Nutmeg (V)
   Fruit of a tree, closely related to the pear tree which came
   originally from the Moluccas and the Sunda Islands.
NUX VOMICA 5c: Nux vomica (V)
   The seed of a shrub from India and Sri Lanka
PODOPHYLLUM 15c: Podophyllum (V)
   The rhizome of a North American plant
PULSATILLA 5c: Meadow anemone (V)
   The whole plant is picked when flowering, in April and
   May. Found in sandy soil throughout Europe.
RHUS TOXICODENDRON 7c: Poison-ivy (V)
   The leaves of a North American and European shrub.
ROBINA 5c: False Acacia (V)
SILICEA 9c: Silica (M)
STRAMONIUM 15c: Thorn-apple (V)
   The whole plant is picked before the flowers bloom in July.
   Grows on rubble-strewn sites and along road verges.
SUFUR IODATUM 5c: Sulphur iodide (M)

TABACUM 5c: Tobacco (V)
Fresh leaves are gathered before the flowers develop in summer.
TARENTULA HISPANA 5c: Tarantula (A)
Spider from the Taranto region of Italy.
VERATRUM ALBUM 5c: White hellebore (V)
The fresh root is gathered at the beginning of June. It is closely related to the colchicum which grows in high mountain pastures.

CLASSIFYING YOUR REMEDIES

Always have ready to hand:
Aconite, Apis, Arnica

Use quickly, frequently indicated:
Allium cepa, Belladona, Cantharis, Chamomilla, Ferrum phosphoricum, Gelsemium, Ignatia, Ipeca, Mercurius solubilis, Nux vomica, Pulsatilla, Pyrogenium, Rhus toxicodendron, Sulfur iodatum, Veratrum album.

It is possible to wait for:
Ambra grisea, Anacardium, Antimonium crudum, Arsenic album, Bryonia, Caesium, Calcarea phosphorica, Chelidonium, China, Cimicifuga, Cocculus, Dulcamara, Euphrasia, Hydrastis, Hyoscyamus, Kali bromatum, Kali carbonicum, Kali phosphoricum, Lycopodium, Nux moschata, Podophyllum, Robinia, Silicea, Stramonium, Tabacum, Tarentula.